Everything You Need to Know to Have a Healthy Twin Pregnancy

Gila Leiter, M.D.

with Rachel Kranz

A Dell Trade Paperback

A DELL TRADE PAPERBACK

Published by
Dell Publishing
a division of
Random House, Inc.
New York, New York

Copyright © 2000 by Gila Leiter, M.D., and Rachel Kranz
Illustrations copyright © 2000 by Jackie Aher
Cover design by Rich Rossiter
Cover photos © 2000 by Penny Gentieu

Dell books may be purchased for business or promotional use or for special sales. For information please write to: Special Markets Department, Random House, Inc., 1540 Broadway, New York, N.Y. 10036.

DTP and the colophon are trademarks of Random House, Inc.

Library of Congress Cataloging-in-Publication Data

Leiter, Gila.
    Everything you need to know to have a healthy twin
pregnancy / Gila Leiter with Rachel Kranz.
       p.   cm.
    Includes index.
    ISBN 978-0-440-50878-6
       1. Multiple pregnancy—popular works. I. Kranz,
    Rachel. II. Title.
RG567 .L45 2000
618.2'5—dc21   00-031471

Book design by Ellen Cipriano

Printed in the United States of America

Published simultaneously in Canada

November 2000

Everything You Need to Know to Have a Healthy Twin Pregnancy

*To my husband Jim Lavin: without his selfless support for
this project it would not have come to fruition.*

*To Yonit, Sarah, Talia, and Leore, our four beautiful daughters, who
fill every day with joy, love, and on-the-job training.*

*To my patients, especially the brave mothers of multiples, who have
been eager to see this book in print.*

Acknowledgments

I want to thank my colleagues Dr. Sheldon Cherry and Dr. Joanne Stone, who carefully reviewed this manuscript and made important suggestions. Suzanne Coleman, MS, RNC, and Elinor Klein had excellent insights and I'm grateful for their time. Sharon Friedman helped me realize this dream, even in the midst of a cross-continent move. My editor Danielle Perez has been a delight to work with, and her skill and enthusiasm is greatly appreciated. And finally, I want to thank Rachel Kranz, a gifted writer, who has become a dear friend.

Contents

Introduction:
Why This Book–
A Personal Look

When I found myself pregnant with what I thought would be my second child, I was a practicing obstetrician/gynecologist at a busy private practice in New York City with a growing number of multiple births under our care. I've always enjoyed caring for pregnancies and deliveries of multiples, with their higher rate of prenatal problems and potentially difficult deliveries—there's always something unexpected to deal with. And I have always felt a special sympathy and awe for multiple moms. In any case, I always seemed to be the doctor on call when a set of twins was ready to deliver.

Imagine my surprise, then, when I found that I myself was pregnant with twins. Although as a doctor I was an expert in the field, as a woman I wanted the same comfort and reassurance that every expectant mother is looking for.

Of course, I had access to the latest in medical literature—but like any expectant mother, I wanted to read something more personal. As I did during my first pregnancy, I went looking for a "regular" pregnancy book. Only this time I wanted a pregnancy book about twins.

I found so little to answer my needs! I am a doctor, so at least I had access to other information. But, I thought, what about all the mothers out there who *aren't* doctors? My patients wanted more information than I could give them in an office visit, more than the standard few pages that most pregnancy books devote to the special needs of the twin pregnancy. I vowed that someday I would write a book for them, to share my professional and personal experience. This book is the result of that promise.

The Special Needs of "Multiple Moms"

Any pregnancy, delivery, and motherhood is challenging. But multiple moms know that their experience is demanding in a way that no "singleton" mother could possibly imagine. As writer Betsy Israel put it in her 1998 article in *The New York Times Magazine,* "[M]others of twins, triplets, quadruplets, quintuplets . . . will suggest that I, a mere mother of 'singletons,' *don't have a clue.* We may all be moms but we do not belong to the same national chapter of motherhood."

What are some of the special needs of multiple moms? As the mother of twins, triplets, or quads, you'll be at far greater risk of preterm labor and premature delivery. You'll face a far higher incidence of prenatal complications, and you'll be more likely to have to take early leave from work or even to be treated with bed rest. You may face physical complications from the added strain of carrying additional weight for a longer period of time, and you might feel some extra psychological stress over wondering how you'll feed and care for two or more babies at the same time.

You also have special needs with regard to diet, nutrition, and exercise. You should have more testing and monitoring during pregnancy and delivery. You may face a more complicated delivery, with a greater chance of cesarean section. And you might face special challenges in involving your partner, other children, extended family, and friends in a physically and emotionally demanding experience. But what a great reward at the end of the road!

Coming to Terms with Multiples

If you've just found out that you're going to have twins, triplets, or quads—or if you're considering any form of fertility treatment or Assisted Reproductive Technology (ART)—you're likely to be wondering how you can handle the medical, physical, and psychological challenges. This book is geared to help you through. You might be a career woman in her 40s wondering about how you can balance the demands of your job with the very special needs of a multiple pregnancy. Or you might be the mother of two or three children concerned about caring for their needs as you gain 40 or 50 pounds and are instructed to avoid heavy lifting. Maybe you're in your early 20s, wondering how you and your partner will ever pay for *two* sets of baby clothes, *two* cribs, *two* sets of doctor bills. Perhaps you had ART after years of infertility, longing for one child—but were never prepared for the possibility that you might have two, three, or four at the same time.

Perhaps this is your first pregnancy, and you're wondering what to expect. Maybe this is your first *multiple* pregnancy, and you're asking yourself how this time will be different. Possibly you have a sister, aunt, mother, or girlfriend who's had twins, triplets, or quads, but maybe—even with the recent explosion in multiple births—you're the only multiple mom you know.

This book is your resource. In it, you'll hear not only my voice but also the voices of my patients, as we share with you both my medical knowledge and our personal experience of this very special kind of pregnancy and birth. (The stories here are composites, representing the concerns and experiences that I've observed in my years of private practice.)

We'll start at the beginning—how fertility treatments increase your chances of conceiving multiples (Chapter 1), what you can do to ensure a safe pregnancy *before* getting pregnant (Chapter 2), and the basic biology of multiple conception (Chapter 3). We'll go on to help you explore the many feelings that often accompany a multiple pregnancy, offering you some concrete suggestions for working through the hopes, fears, and fantasies that might come up and some specific ideas for nurturing yourself (Chapter 4). We'll help you choose the doctor who is right for you, as we review the various options of an ob/gyn, a perinatologist, a twin clinic, and a midwife (Chapter 5).

Then I'll proceed to the many medical decisions you'll be making: the hard choices that often come with a twin diagnosis and a thorough review of the tests you might have (Chapter 6), along with a comprehensive look at your diet (Chapter 7), use of medications (Chapter 8), and relationship to work, bed rest, and exercise (Chapter 9). We'll go through your pregnancy trimester by trimester (Chapters 10, 11, and 12), as I review what is happening to your body, what you and your doctor will be discussing, and how your babies are developing. My patients and I will be sharing our own experiences and suggestions throughout.

I'll also talk you through some of the common and uncommon complications of a multiple pregnancy, including a look at how diabetes might affect you and your babies (Chapter 13). We'll take a long look at the possibility of preterm labor and premature delivery (Chapters 14 and 15), which pose the greatest risk to the life and health of multiple babies and which you and your doctor will be making every effort to avoid.

Finally, I'll talk you through the birthing process, explaining the kinds of decisions you and your doctor might have to make (Chapter 16) and giving you a blow-by-blow description of what you might expect in the delivery room, including the possibility of a breech birth or C-section (Chapter 17). You'll hear about those first few days in the hospital (Chapter 18) and find out what it's like to bring your multiples home (Chapter 19). At the end of this book, there's a list of resources—Web sites, books, and organizations—that might help you through your pregnancy and early years as the parents of twins.

As I review this chapter, I'm sitting on the labor floor at Mt. Sinai Hospital, taking a welcome break after finishing my morning rounds. I've got two sets of twins on the postpartum floor: one that was delivered very early, at 27 weeks, due to the mother's complication of *placenta previa* (a condition in which the placenta covers part of the cervix); another that stayed in the womb for a full 37-week term. Thanks to the miracles of modern science, all four babies are doing well, and both mothers are recovering nicely. I continue to marvel at how bravely and gracefully my patients manage the many challenges and surprises of a multiple pregnancy—and at the joy and excitement that a multiple birth can bring.

Preventing Prematurity: Your Number-One Goal

One of the most important objectives of your multiple pregnancy can be expressed very simply: *to carry your babies to term.*

This is not as simple as it may sound. A multiple pregnancy is far more likely than a singleton to end in preterm labor and premature delivery—with consequent risks to your babies. As a pregnant multiple mom, you need to do everything you can to prolong your pregnancy—eat right, avoid certain types of exertion, follow your doctor's orders with regard to lifestyle, work life, and bed rest.

If your babies are born prematurely, you want them to come into the world as big and strong as possible, to compensate for the problems caused by early delivery. So you also need to eat right from the very beginning of your pregnancy to ensure early, adequate weight gain.

Much of what I discuss in this book is geared toward helping you have the healthiest babies you can by making the very most of their time in the womb. As I'll be repeating many times before the book is done: Knowledge is power. While you can't have complete control over when your babies "decide" to come out, you can do a great deal to promote their health and safety.

Exploring the Mystery of Twins

"Everyone is interested in twins—or they should be," wrote Horatio H. Newman, an early student of twins, and certainly most societies that we know of have shown a remarkable fascination with twins and other multiples. Twin lore goes back to ancient times. In the Bible, for example, Jacob and Esau were twins, as were Zarah and Pharez, the father of King David, while Greek mythology features such twins as Apollo the sun god and Artemis the moon goddess.

It's not only Western mythology that reveals this fascination with twins. In most cultures, pregnancy and birth are themselves seen as mysterious and thrilling—and multiple births seem even more so. In some societies, twins are viewed as a kind of punishment; in others, they are seen as a divine reward bestowed upon the parents. Most of the multiple moms I know, myself included, feel that both are true.

Twins are frequently the subjects in scientific studies that seek to establish the boundaries between "nature" and "nurture," especially with monozygotic (popularly called "identical") twins separated at birth. Certainly, in my own experience as a New York City ob/gyn, I've seen that multiple moms enjoy a certain honor, a special kind of respect and wonder. When a woman pregnant with twins walks into our waiting room, there's a kind of hush that falls over the room. Even other pregnant women are a bit in awe. And whenever we deliver twins or triplets, even in a delivery room where everyone is more or less used to "the miracle of birth," there's a way that the whole labor floor holds its breath and then bursts into applause when the multiples arrive.

A Growing Number of "Multiple Moms"

In the ten years since I had my own twin daughters, the number of multiple moms has risen at an extraordinary rate, and 1 in 40 births in the United States is twins. This statistical increase is being reflected more and more often in popular culture. *The New York Times Sunday Magazine, The New Yorker,* and numerous other journals have published articles on twins, triplets, quads, and other multiple births. TV news programs focus on famous quints, sextuplets, or octuplets; TV movies explore the joys and sorrows of multiple parenthood. A casual walk through the streets of your own neighborhood will reveal more double strollers and identically dressed babies than ever before.

The New Generation of Multiple Moms

Gone are the days when a doctor can respond to a patient's queries by saying dismissively, "Don't worry, dearie, it's just doctor talk"—and I say, good riddance! My patients are a diverse group that includes actresses, professors, and athletes; runway models concerned about keeping their fashionably thin figures; union women on group health plans; professional women who want to know how to manage multiple pregnancies and their careers at the same time; and women who have been eagerly awaiting their pregnancies through several years of infertility treatment. But they all have one thing in common: They all want to know as much as possible about their condition, so that they can work with me to make the best possible choices for themselves and the babies they're carrying.

I couldn't be happier about the new, more confident and assertive attitude that I see among women patients. I want my patients to have access to all the information they need, so they can be more proactive in going through their pregnancies and making decisions about giving birth. I firmly believe that there's no topic that's too esoteric for a lay-person to understand if it's explained well. Even in controversial matters—especially in controversial matters—I'd rather that the patient know as much as possible about the issues. Being informed will only make things better for both her and me—and the babies!

Knowledge Is Power

One of the most exciting things about this period in medical history is the number of areas in which we now know enough to enable pregnant women to make positive interventions in their pregnancy. For example, it has now become clear that taking sufficient quantities of folic acid (vitamin B_{12}) from the moment of conception reduces the risk of neural-tube defects—involved in spina bifida and other conditions—by 75 percent. What a discovery! Just by taking a vitamin supplement while trying to get pregnant, you can go a long way toward ensuring the health of your babies in one important area with little risk and even the possible benefit of reducing your own chances of heart disease and colon cancer later in life.

Yet a recent March of Dimes survey revealed that only 12 percent of pregnant women knew about this finding (although this number seems to be increasing). The knowledge exists—but many women do not have access to it or are not making use of it. The full potential of our recent medical advances is not being reached.

One of my goals for this book is to help every woman who is pregnant with multiples make the best possible use of the most current medical information available. Of course, pregnancy is by its very nature a risky business—and multiple pregnancy even more so. But there are so many ways you can reduce the risks and increase your chances of a safe delivery with happy outcomes all around. Your doctor is one resource in this process. This book is another.

Embarking on Your Journey

Every ob/gyn knows that there is no such thing as only one "normal" pregnancy or delivery. Every expectant mother is unique, every couple is different, and every childbirth has its own logic and outcome. If this is true in general, it goes double for twins! My wish is that this book can provide you with the information, insight, and support that you need to navigate your own unique experience of pregnancy, childbirth, and motherhood.

Everything You Need to Know to Have a Healthy Twin Pregnancy

1.

Fertility Treatments,
Assisted Reproductive Technology,
and Your Chances of Having Twins

Jeannette was a 36-year-old vice president at an investment securities company. She and her husband had been trying to get pregnant for several months, with no success. After undergoing the usual battery of tests, Jeannette went to see a fertility specialist, who prescribed Pergonal, a medication commonly used to promote ovulation.

Within three months, Jeannette and her husband were delighted to learn that they were finally pregnant. But they were both taken aback to discover that theirs was a multiple pregnancy. Like many women undergoing infertility treatments, Jeannette had conceived twins.

ART and Multiple Pregnancies

The number of women conceiving multiple pregnancies has gone up dramatically in the past ten years—and the rate of increase is getting faster every year. About one-third of the marked upswing in multiple pregnancies is due to the fact that these days, many women don't even start trying to get pregnant until they're between the ages of 35 and

39—statistically, the most likely ages for a woman to conceive twins or other multiples.

However, the other two-thirds of the increase in multiple gestations is due to fertility treatments. Studies have shown that 37 percent of all live births that resulted from "assisted reproductive techniques" were multiple births. *That means that if you're having any form of fertility treatment or ART, your chances of getting pregnant with twins, triplets, quads, or quints is more than 1 in 3.*

Of course, the two factors are connected. If you're trying to conceive after the age of 35, it may take you longer—and, like Jeannette, you might be tempted to turn to ART sooner than a younger woman would. ART is a wonderful invention that has helped lots of women bear the children that they want—but it does also carry with it a vastly increased likelihood of giving birth to twins, triplets, and other multiples.

ART and Multiple Pregnancies

The number of women using ART is going up all the time. According to a study sponsored by the Society for Assisted Reproductive Technology, the American Society for Reproductive Medicine, and the Centers for Disease Control and Prevention, the number of ART procedures conducted between 1994 and 1995 rose by almost 20 percent. Most couples having ART were undergoing *in vitro fertilization* (IVF), though a variety of other methods—*gamete intrafallopian transfers* (GIFT), *zygote intrafallopian transfers, frozen-embryo thaw procedures,* and *donor oocyte cycles,* among others—were also used.

The incidence of twins, triplets, and higher-order multiples represents about 1 to 2 percent of all pregnancies. If you're having ART, however, your chances of conceiving multiples are far higher: for twins, 25 to 30 percent, for triplets, 5 to 6 percent, for quads or higher-order multiples, 0.5 to 1 percent. In other words, some 35 to 50 percent of all twins born recently, and over 77 percent of recent higher-order births, are the result of some sort of infertility therapy.

When Jeannette learned these statistics, she understood a bit more about how her twin pregnancy had transpired. Unfortunately, she didn't find out about her increased chances of conceiving multiples

The Dramatic Increase in Multiple Pregnancies

- The natural incidence of twins is 1 in 89—but in the past few decades, thanks to ovulation induction, Assisted Reproductive Technology (ART), and other interventions, the birth rate of twins in the United States has jumped to 1 in 40!
- In other words, since 1980, the rate of twins has risen 37 percent.
- Also since 1980, the rate of triplets and higher-order multiples has increased 312 percent.
- Between 1995 and 1996 alone, the rate of triplets jumped 19 percent.
- In 1996, nearly 6,000 babies were born in triplets, quads, or even larger sets of multiple births—and experts expect that number to keep going up.

until after the fact. When she came to me, Jeannette had decidedly mixed feelings about her experience with fertility treatment.

"I guess I had some vague sense that *some* women got pregnant with twins when they took fertility drugs," she told me. "But I had no idea that the figures were so high. My husband and I are overjoyed that we're finally pregnant—and we've just about adjusted to the idea that it's twins. But what if we'd had triplets, or even quads? I wish I'd known more before we started the whole process."

Although we may someday have better control over the outcomes of fertility treatment and ART, women who are currently undergoing such treatment should not be surprised to find themselves carrying more than one baby. So if you're having or considering fertility treatment, I advise you to work closely with your doctor or fertility specialist to learn the latest data on the method you're using. Find out your chances of conceiving twins, triplets, or other multiples—and weigh your feelings about a multiple pregnancy against your wish to be pregnant.

How Fertility Treatment Works

Why is fertility treatment causing this explosion of multiple pregnancies? Let's take a closer look.

There are two basic ways that doctors can help an infertile couple to conceive:

1. *Fertility medications.* Most fertility drugs cause superovulation, boosting fertility by increasing the available number of eggs. But the more eggs available, the greater the chances that more than one will be fertilized—resulting in twins, triplets, quads, or more. Women who take the popular fertility medication Clomid have an 8 percent chance of conceiving twins. Jeannette, who had been prescribed Pergonal, another medication that promotes ovulation, had a 20 to 40 percent chance of conceiving twins.

2. *In vitro fertilization (IVF).* In addition to boosting the number of eggs, a couple may choose to ensure that the eggs are fertilized. Rather than relying upon natural fertilization—the father's sperm reaching the mother's egg during intercourse—IVF boosts the chances of conception by harvesting the eggs and having them fertilized in vitro—in a glass dish. One or more fertilized eggs are then transferred back into the mother's uterus, where hopefully she carries at least one of them to term. This is a technique that must be used if the woman's tubes are blocked, if there are problems with the man's fertility, or if there's unexplained infertility or endometriosis.

A common variation of IVF is known as ICSI: *intracytoplasmic sperm injection.* In this technique, the sperm is injected directly into the egg. This method makes it possible for men with even very low sperm counts to father children.

Still, with either IVF or ICSI, one tricky decision immediately presents itself: How many embryos should be transplanted back into the mother? Obviously, choosing just one embryo eliminates the possibility of a multiple pregnancy—but if that embryo does not survive, the whole cycle must begin again. On the other hand, transplanting, say, five embryos raises the possibility of quintuplets—unlikely, to be sure, but as recent headlines have demonstrated, not impossible. Certainly, transferring five embryos is more likely to result in twins or even triplets than transferring only one embryo.

The IVF Controversy

As the increased use of IVF has led to an increase in multiple pregnancies, a controversy has arisen over the way IVF is conducted. Should doctors transfer as many fertilized embryos as possible back into the mother? This increases the chances of her getting pregnant—but also increases her chances of a multiple pregnancy.

A similar controversy reigns with the use of fertility medicines like Pergonal and Clomid. Prescribed in higher doses, they are more likely to stimulate greater egg production in the mother—increasing both her chances for pregnancy in general and her likelihood of conceiving twins, triplets, or quads.

Another approach is to establish checkpoints, whereby the doctor monitors how many eggs are released in each cycle. That way, a woman can use birth control or avoid intercourse if too many eggs become available. Again, however, this more conservative approach also reduces the chances of *any* pregnancy.

Meanwhile, infertile couples face a number of pressures to choose stronger fertility drugs and more aggressive treatments. For example, limited health-insurance coverage for infertility treatments leads many couples to feel that they must get pregnant quickly, even if they conceive twins, triplets, or quads in the process.

In the wake of adverse publicity about quads and quints, the United Kingdom, Belgium, Germany, Australia, and Singapore have actually passed laws limiting the number of embryos that can be transferred back into the uterus at each IVF cycle. Many U.S. doctors think that we should have similar laws in this country—though other physicians point out that such regulation runs counter to the U.S. tradition of free choice in medicine and privately regulated health care.

What Can Be Done?

Certainly, laws or no laws, doctors can—and should—take steps to reduce the chances of a multiple pregnancy. In the case of fertility medications, a doctor can monitor the number of ripe eggs that become available during the cycle. If too many eggs are available in a particular month, the doctor can advise the patient to terminate the cycle.

In Jeannette's case, for example, the Pergonal evidently caused two eggs to ripen, leading to her pregnancy with twins. Potentially, the medication could have led to the release of three or even four eggs. If Jeannette and her husband had strong feelings about *not* conceiving multiples, they might have chosen to avoid pregnancy that particular month.

What about women who are using IVF? In those cases, doctors should be very careful in deciding how many embryos to transfer into a woman's uterus, based on the woman's age, her history of fertility, and other factors that affect her ability to carry one or more babies to term.

We're continually learning more about how to weigh the benefits of pregnancy against the risks of a multiple conception. For example, a 1998 study published in *Fertility and Sterility,* the journal of the American Society for Reproductive Medicine, suggests that the number of embryos most likely to produce a singleton pregnancy varies based on the woman's age and on the quality of the embryo. (The "quality" of the embryo refers to its chances of survival.) The study's authors came up with the following recommendations:

- For women 35 and under, transfer either four poor-quality, two fair-quality, or two good-quality embryos.
- For women ages 36 to 39, transfer four poor-quality, three fair-quality, or two good-quality embryos.
- For women age 40 or over, transfer five embryos *regardless of embryo quality.*

A 1996 *Fertility and Sterility* article found that for women under the age of 34, transferring more than two or three embryos increased the risk of multiple pregnancy without actually increasing the chances of pregnancy. The study's authors felt that for women under age 34, no more than three embryos should be transferred—possibly fewer, as doctors improve their ability to preselect only those embryos with the best chances of survival.

Balancing the Decision

As you can see, different couples require different approaches. Older couples, for example, or those who have not responded well to previous fertility treatments may need a more aggressive fertility treatment—with more risk of a multiple pregnancy.

Younger couples, on the other hand, or couples who are just beginning fertility treatments might want to be more conservative in their approach. They may need to accept, however, that such an approach could take longer and involve greater expense—not to mention greater disappointment.

Of course, some couples actively welcome the possibility of twins and triplets. However, given the increased medical risks and the greater costs of a multiple pregnancy, a couple may need to consider a more cautious approach. Yes, an "instant family" might be nice—but there are tremendous health risks, emotional costs, and financial expenses involved.

Still other couples are willing to undergo aggressive fertility treatments with the expectation that, if triplets, quads, or a higher-order pregnancy results, they'll "reduce" it: that is, they'll abort one or more of the multiples, either for health reasons or to keep their family small. However, some patients, doctors, and hospitals won't consider reduction or will consider it only for reasons of health, especially since reduction brings some (small) risk to the entire pregnancy.

Finally, some couples might be deeply committed to avoiding a multiple pregnancy—for health reasons, financial considerations, personal preferences, or some combination of the above. These couples may decide against using ART at all—even if it means they never get pregnant.

Making Your Decision

Clearly, if you're undergoing fertility treatments of any kind, your doctor needs to know about your preferences. How would *you* balance your wish to get pregnant quickly with your wish to avoid a multiple pregnancy? Here are some questions you need to ask in order to make your decision:

- **How likely is a given fertility treatment to be successful, given your medical history?** Older couples, couples with poor baseline hormone levels, or couples with a long history of infertility may have more difficulty becoming pregnant unless the fertility treatment is "stepped up" to a level that is more likely to produce multiples.
- **Are you willing to consider ovum (egg) donation?** One way for older or less fertile couples to increase their chances of pregnancy without a higher risk of multiples is to use another woman's eggs, which may be easier to fertilize with a less aggressive treatment. However, the couple then has to be willing to accept another person's genetic material.
- **How likely is a given treatment to produce a multiple pregnancy?** Some fertility medications are more potent than others.
- **What are the costs and risks of a multiple pregnancy?** As we've seen, this answer varies depending on the couple. For couples with high incomes and lots of child-care options, a multiple pregnancy might seem less daunting. For a woman with high blood pressure, diabetes, or other medical conditions, a multiple pregnancy might seem especially risky. And of course, only you and your partner know if you're ready to take on the challenge of parenting two, three, or even more children at the same time.

Thinking It Through

At this point in our medical knowledge, I think that anyone who's considering infertility treatment with ovulation induction must be prepared for the possibility of a multiple pregnancy. And anyone who's undergoing ART needs to work with her doctor to weigh not conceiving at all against conceiving twins, triplets, or even quads.

For example, another one of my patients, Sandra, had gotten pregnant with IVF, only to deliver prematurely at 28 weeks. The second time she used IVF, she had an early miscarriage at 8 weeks. So when her next treatment with IVF led to her pregnancy with twins, she had two reasons to be concerned: Both her previous history and the fact of her multiple pregnancy put her at special risk of preterm labor. Ideally, the doctors who did her IVF procedure would have been especially careful to avoid higher-order multiples, since that was likely to be a particularly risky pregnancy for her. (Fortunately, after intense monitoring and bed rest, she had a fairly long pregnancy and delivered her healthy twins at 34 weeks.)

Another patient, Ally, suffered from ulcerative colitis and had undergone multiple surgeries on her bowel, which led to adhesions. When she used ART to get pregnant, she was especially concerned about the possibility of conceiving multiples, since her previous surgical history had already put her at risk for a C-section. (In her case, the ART resulted in a singleton pregnancy.)

The good news is that we're learning more about fertility every day, and our techniques for IVF are improving rapidly. I think that the trend of transferring fewer healthy embryos, at a later stage of their development, will become more common and will thus allow us to lower the risk for multiple pregnancies. In my opinion, this is the wave of the future.

2.

How Can I Prepare for Having Twins?

M y patient Rosario had just started trying to get pregnant, and she was taking the process quite seriously. She came into my office one day with a long list of questions about what to eat, what vitamins and supplements to take, what exercises would help her get into shape for the delivery, and whether it was okay to take aspirin for an occasional headache. Then she asked a question that I wish more prospective mothers would ask: "What *else* do I need to know, Dr. Leiter? What questions should I be asking that I haven't even thought of?"

Touching All the Bases: A Look at Your Personal Situation

You already know that you'll need to take care of your babies while they're in your womb. But in the last ten years, we've learned quite a bit about an even earlier stage of prenatal planning—the care that begins before your babies are even conceived. Known as *preconception* or *prepregnancy* care, this approach is based on the notion that you'll want all your physical and emotional resources in place to cope with the demands of carrying a child and giving birth. And that goes double— or even triple!—for a multiple pregnancy.

Also, many of the factors in your environment, family history, or medical condition that might cause problems with being pregnant can also interfere with *getting* pregnant. So looking closely at your health, history, and surroundings is helpful all around.

Those First Eight Weeks

In your babies' first two months of life, they're forming their organ systems and just beginning to grow. So they're more vulnerable than they'll ever be again to infections, alcohol, drugs, and environmental hazards. Yet you might not even realize that you *are* pregnant until some or all of this early time has passed.

In either case, as soon as you start trying to get pregnant, you should probably act as though you're already carrying one or two fetuses. Start by talking to your doctor.

Your Preconception Exam

Ideally, you and the baby's father-to-be should each have a complete physical exam at least three months before you stop using birth control. This has a double purpose: You can address conditions that might be harmful to you or the baby during pregnancy, and you can identify problems that might interfere with your or the father's fertility.

What to Expect at Your Preconception Exam

- A complete history and physical.
- An updated Pap smear.
- Tests—with your and your partner's permission—for any sexually transmitted diseases and for the HIV virus. (Mothers infected with any of these diseases face special problems during pregnancy and delivery, and they won't be able to breast-feed. The good news is that treating the mom with antiviral agents can dramatically reduce her chance of transmitting HIV to her baby.)
- A CBC—or complete blood count—to check for anemia and other conditions that might affect pregnancy and delivery.

- Tests to find out if you have been exposed to certain conditions (see below).
- A discussion of your medications for any ongoing medical problems, such as asthma, thyroid disease, diabetes, a heart defect, high blood pressure, or depression. Your doctor may want to change your meds, or you might be advised to delay getting pregnant until your condition is under better control.
- A discussion of your family history and ethnic background to help the doctor decide what kind of screening you might need for ethnically linked genetic conditions (see below). Prepare for this discussion by finding out as much as possible about your and your partner's family background: What ethnic groups are represented? What medical conditions run in either family? Is there any history of mental retardation or birth defects?

Of course, you and your ob/gyn will need to have a full discussion of your health—both your general and your gynecological health—once you actually do become pregnant. But your doctor should know as much as possible ahead of time, to alert you to concerns you might not have anticipated. Here are some questions that your doctor might ask:

- Do you have an abnormal uterine shape or uterine fibroids?
- Have you got an enlarged thyroid or hirsutism (a hormonal condition that results in the unusual growth of body hair)?
- Do you have any history of blood clots? A decreased number of blood platelets? Any experience of anemia?
- What's your menstrual history?
- Have you ever been pregnant, including ectopic (tubal) pregnancies?
- Did you ever bleed during pregnancy? How much and which trimester?
- Do you have any history with preterm labor or premature delivery?
- If you have given birth, how long did you carry each baby, and how big was he or she?

If You Have a History of Miscarriage . . .

Most miscarriages are due to genetic abnormalities in the fetus, which won't necessarily be a factor in the next pregnancy. Sometimes, though, miscarriage is caused by hormonal factors or by various types of undiagnosed auto-immune conditions. Occasionally a miscarriage may be caused by infection or by some kind of anatomic disorder. If you do have a history of miscarriages, your doctor may test you for one or more of these conditions as you try to become pregnant.

- Have you ever lost a pregnancy? A woman who has already had two miscarriages faces an increased risk of miscarriage with each subsequent pregnancy—although the risk is somewhat less if the woman has carried full-term pregnancies as well. The good news is that even after three losses without treatment, a woman can hope to deliver a healthy baby at least 50 percent of the time. Of course, any woman who *has* lost a pregnancy should be monitored closely, to make sure that the baby's growth is normal and to watch for preterm labor.

Testing Your Immunity

One of the questions Rosario forgot to ask was whether she had immunity to various common conditions that might cause birth defects or other problems during pregnancy. Ideally, you'll ask this question *before* you get pregnant, since there are many immunizations you can't have once you're carrying a child. Your doctor will want to know if you're at risk for infections like the following:

- **Rubella (German measles)**—If you're not already immune, there's a vaccine for this. But you shouldn't get pregnant for at least three months after you've been vaccinated, since the vaccine causes you to secrete live virus. (As I was writing this, a recent rubella outbreak in the affluent suburban county of Westchester, New York, underscored the importance of vaccinating at-risk women.)

- **Chicken pox**—Some 80 percent of all women carry antibodies to this common childhood disease, mainly because they had chicken pox when they were children. A history of chicken pox is a reliable indication that you're immune. If you've never had chicken pox, you should get an antibody titer—a test of the levels of the chicken pox antibody in your bloodstream. The odds are that you'll still be immune, even if you don't remember having the disease. If you test negative, though, ask your doctor about being vaccinated, since getting chicken pox in your first trimester could cause birth defects.
- **Toxoplasmosis**—This parasitic infection can be picked up from changing the cat's litter box (although it's rare in housebound cats), gardening without gloves, or eating raw or undercooked meat. You might be immune to this condition, but if you're not sure, avoid these activities while pregnant or trying to get pregnant.
- **Hepatitis B**—You're at risk of this liver disease if you work in a health-care facility or handle blood products. If you do carry the hep B virus, you've got about a 50 percent chance of passing it on to your babies—putting them at risk of developing liver damage or cancer later in life. If you're likely to come in contact with hepatitis B, you should have a series of vaccines before trying to get pregnant.

Get in Shape!

It's difficult to get into good physical condition after you become pregnant, particularly with twins, triplets, or quads. So ideally you'll give yourself time to get into excellent physical shape before you actually conceive. If you can, commit to:

- regular aerobic exercise;
- stretching exercises that keep your muscles toned and flexible;

If You Have a Chronic Condition . . .

Certain conditions pose special risks during pregnancy: diabetes, hypertension, some types of arthritis, anemia, thyroid conditions, asthma, and systemic lupus erythematosus (SLE). If you have any one of these—or if there's a family history of these conditions—tell your physician, since you might be facing special risks during pregnancy and delivery.

For example, diabetes and thyroid disease increase the rate of miscarriage. Endocrine factors such as polycystic ovarian syndrome (PCOs) might affect your hormone levels and keep you from ovulating regularly, which can also interfere with fertility and increase your risk of miscarriage. Maternal thyroid disease can result in learning problems for the offspring, so many ob/gyns are screening for this condition before and in early pregnancy.

If you've got a chronic condition of any kind, try to get pregnant when your condition is "optimized." For example, if you have ulcerative colitis that has ever required surgery, your pregnancy will go better if you conceive while in remission than when you're acutely ill. And a woman with poorly controlled diabetes is four to six times more likely to have a baby with birth defects than a woman without diabetes. On the other hand, a woman whose blood sugars are well controlled before and during pregnancy has almost the same chance to have a healthy baby as the woman without diabetes.

None of these conditions means you *can't* get pregnant. But check with your doctor about the best precautions to take. Being informed can help you protect your baby's health!

- back exercises, which will vastly ease the process of labor and delivery (for suggestions, see Chapter 9).

By the way, women who start exercising several months before getting pregnant tend to have easier pregnancies and deliveries than women who are not so physically fit. And, as with many aspects of pregnancy, that's even more true for multiple moms.

Weight

One of the things that most worried Rosario was her weight, since she was about 20 pounds heavier than was ideal for her size. Ironically, another one of my patients, Shana, was a runway model who was 20 pounds underweight—and *she* wasn't concerned at all. In fact, both women were running certain risks.

Underweight women often have a harder time conceiving than other prospective mothers. And when they do get pregnant, especially with multiples, they have to make a special effort to eat right during the first few weeks of pregnancy in order to guarantee their babies' early, adequate weight gain. (For more on this topic, see Chapter 7.)

On the other hand, very obese women (those who weigh at least 25 percent more than their ideal body weights) may face increased risk of birth defects, late-term fetal death, and the death of babies born prematurely. Since many multiples *are* born prematurely, obesity is a special concern for multiple moms.

In my experience, most women tend to think they're heavier than they are. Even Rosario, who did need to lose some weight, didn't need to lose as much as she *thought* she did. And of course, starvation diets and excessive exercise tend to decrease ovulation.

So remember—moderation in all things! Basically, you want a diet-and-exercise plan that will improve your conditioning, strength, and lean body mass—not a regime aimed at making you supermodel-thin. Work with your doctor to develop the healthy eating habits—including eating enough protein and calcium—and to find the exercise routines that will stand you in good stead both before and during pregnancy.

Supplements

One of the best things you can do for your baby is to take at least 0.4 daily milligrams of folic acid from the moment you conceive (in addition to eating foods rich in this nutrient, such as leafy green vegetables, orange juice, and beans). Practically speaking, that means that you should start taking this supplement from the moment you start trying to get pregnant. Folic acid seems to make a dramatic difference in decreasing the incidence of neural-tube defects such as spina bifida. In fact, if you're at a high risk for bearing a child with a neural-tube defect (talk to your doctor), you'll want to take 4 mg of this amazing supplement each day.

Once you conceive, you'll want to take a pregnancy multivitamin, and possibly supplement with iron and calcium as well. There are also some vitamin and mineral supplements that you'll want to avoid. (For more information on supplements, see Chapter 8.) Meanwhile, be sure that while you're trying to get pregnant, your diet includes plenty of protein, calcium, iron, vitamins, and minerals.

Smoking

If you're a smoker, or if you live with a smoker, this prepregnancy time is an excellent occasion to consider the health hazards of smoking and of secondhand smoke for the unborn children you may carry:

- Both direct and secondhand smoke (smoke inhaled from someone else's cigarette) are associated with low birth weight. As we'll see throughout this book, low birth weight is of particular concern to parents of multiples, since twins, triplets, and quads are already likely to be born at lower birth weights than singletons. So anything you can do to increase your children's birth weight can make a crucial difference to their lives and their health.
- Both direct and secondhand smoke are associated with a rate of miscarriage as much as two times higher than that of the general population.
- Some evidence suggests that sudden infant death syndrome (SIDS) is more likely to occur in homes where somebody smokes.
- Some doctors believe that babies born to mothers who smoke— or who are exposed to large amounts of secondary smoke—have a slower growth rate and do less well on IQ tests than they otherwise would.
- The mother's exposure to secondhand smoke has actually been known to cause asthma and other lung diseases in unborn children.

What does this mean for you? Simply put: If you smoke, stop before you become pregnant. If someone in your household smokes, enlist that person's commitment to creating a smoke-free atmosphere for
you while you are pregnant and for your children after they are born.

What about smoking at work or in social situations? This was a
concern for Jeannette: Although technically her workplace was supposed to be a smoke-free zone, her boss was a chain smoker who felt
entitled to exercise his habit in the privacy of his office. Even though
he courteously abstained from smoking whenever Jeannette was actually there, she could feel her throat drying out from the smoke that
remained in the air during their frequent conferences.

Jeannette agonized over how to handle the situation. "I had already asked for maternity leave," she says, "and I hated to call any extra
attention to myself as a woman. I'd worked hard to get where I was—
to *not* be seen as 'the woman who needed special treatment'—but
now I *did* need special treatment. I was willing to risk my own health
every time I went into my boss's office—but I didn't want to put my
babies at risk."

Finally, Jeannette decided that her babies' health was more important to her than any other consideration. She asked her boss if they
could meet in the smoke-free conference room while she was pregnant. "I don't think he was crazy about the idea," she told me. "And I
do think he sees me differently now. I hope I can make up for that
now that the babies are born—but I still think it was worth it."

Drinking and Drugs

Drinking and recreational drugs are also associated with enormous
prenatal risks. If you think you might have any difficulty avoiding alcohol or recreational drugs during your pregnancy, now is the time to
get help.

Even if you don't have a problem with alcohol, you might want to
avoid drinking while you're trying to get pregnant. And drinking
while pregnant might contribute to your child being born with facial
deformities and/or mental retardation at birth, or developing learning
and behavioral difficulties while growing up. Likewise, recreational

The Baby's Father

It's not only you who has to be careful while trying to conceive. Alcohol, to-bacco, marijuana, and other recreational drugs can also affect a man's sperm, making it more difficult to conceive and posing possible problems to the baby if you do get pregnant. It takes about three months to produce sperm, so your baby's father should be "clean" three months before the two of you start trying to conceive.

drugs, even in moderate quantities, also pose problems for fertility as well as fetuses, especially early in the pregnancy.

What About Prescription and Over-the-Counter Drugs?

This is a tricky area, because some drugs pose virtually no risk, while others pose enormous risk—and still others may put you at risk if you *don't* take them. If you are currently taking medication for asthma, thyroid disease, colitis, depression, or seizures, you will almost certainly need to take some version of your current medication while you are pregnant.

Of course, the final arbiter will be your physician. But you can get a head start by researching your particular form of medication and possible pregnancy-safe substitutes. There are many excellent resources, including some sites on the Internet, such as Reprotox and Motherisk. (For their addresses and for additional information, see the Resources section of this book.) Ideally, your doctor will prescribe the switch in medications *before* you become pregnant, so you can see how you respond to the new treatment.

Most likely, your doctor will be switching you to older drugs—because we know more about them—while prescribing the smallest possible effective dosage for you. However, it's important for both you and your doctor to keep up to date. For example, Prozac, widely used to treat depression, is newer than some other antidepressants—but is most likely safe for pregnant women. Although some evidence suggests that women on Prozac may experience third-trimester complications, most of the studies done so far show no increase in risk from this medication.

Over-the-counter drugs are trickier, since most pose at least some risk to your unborn children. When Rosario came to me for prepregnancy counseling, she asked about aspirin (which she took for occasional headaches), over-the-counter cold remedies, nonprescription allergy medication, and an antacid she took for gas and heartburn. I told her the antacid was fine, but that she'd do well to avoid the other medications if she possibly could. She was happy to comply, but if she'd been more concerned, I would have worked with her to come up with some pregnancy-safe substitutes. I suggest that you, too, make a list of the nonprescription drugs you usually take and talk to your doctor about each of them. (For more on medication do's and don't's, see Chapter 8.)

Finally, if you're taking birth-control pills, you should know that most doctors recommend that women have at least two normal periods before trying to get pregnant. That way, normal ovulation will resume and the pregnancy can be dated accurately. However, no study has shown any increased risk if you do become pregnant either while on the pill or shortly after you've stopped taking it.

What's in Your Environment?

Environmental toxins can disrupt your hormones and interfere with your immune system. If you use cleaning products at home, pesticides in your garden, or standard office products at work, you may be exposing yourself to environmental risks. Likewise, you might be endangering your pregnancy if you work in a factory, dry cleaner, plant nursery, or any other workplace where cleaning solvents, industrial chemicals, or pesticides are used. A study by the National Center for Health Statistics found that almost one-fifth of all of working women were exposed to known *teratogens* (substances that cause birth defects) during their pregnancy.

Another common group of toxins is the so-called "heavy metals"—lead, mercury, cadmium, and manganese—which appear variously in water, food, soil, and air. If you live in an old house, you might want to have it tested for lead, used widely in paint for decades before its dangers were known. If you have any concerns about environmental toxins, discuss the risks with your doctor while observing a few basic precautions:

- Make sure you're working in a well-ventilated environment, particularly if you're using cleaning products, paints, pesticides, or solvents.
- If your job involves prolonged exposure to paint, pesticides, or other toxic substances, you might want to make other arrangements during your pregnancy.
- Cross-country flying up until the 20th week of pregnancy is fine on an occasional basis, but pilots, flight attendants, and women who travel frequently on business should consult Federal Aviation Authority (FAA) guidelines, as certain routes—particularly those close to the poles—expose you to greater radiation from the sun.

Many of my patients ask me about hair dye, microwaves, and computer screens. Fortunately, these are all perfectly safe.

Your Family History

Besides knowing about *your* obstetrical history, your doctor will want to know about your family. Start by finding out as much as you can about the pregnancies and obstetrical histories of your mother, sisters, and mother's mother. Were their deliveries easy or difficult? Did any of them deliver early or go into preterm labor? Does your family have any history of twinning—especially dizygotic twinning—or of other multiple pregnancies?

Your and your partner's family histories may also reveal genetic issues. Unfortunately, there is no one test that both you and your partner can take to detect all risk of genetic disease. Some genetic diseases are associated with particular ethnic groups; others tend to run in families.

Get Ready to Get Pregnant!

- Eat a well-balanced diet full of calcium, iron, and protein.
- Take at least 0.4 milligrams of folic acid a day.
- Get some exercise, such as walking or swimming, several times a week.
- Try to achieve a reasonable weight for your height.
- Go with the baby's father to get tested for STDs.
- Get vaccinated against any infections for which you're at risk.
- Review all prescription and over-the-counter medications with your doctor—including your birth-control pills and your use of aspirin, cold medication, and so on.
- Make sure that any long-term health problems—diabetes, a heart condition, blood pressure, asthma—are under control.
- Stop using alcohol, recreational drugs, and nicotine.
- Take care of any medical or dental work that requires X rays.
- Make sure that neither your home nor your workplace is exposing you to radiation, lead, gas fumes, or other environmental toxins.

Ethnically Linked Genetic Conditions

- **Sickle-cell anemia**—This painful condition is most often found among African-Americans and, more rarely, among some Mediterranean groups as well. Abnormally shaped—"sickle-shaped"—cells get stuck in blood vessels, which can cause pain and anemia. Approximately 1 in 10 people with African-American ancestry carries this disease, which is screened for through a blood test known as hemoglobin electrophoresis. Carriers of sickle-cell have a higher rate of urinary tract infections (UTIs), so if you're a carrier, your doctor will probably take monthly urine cultures.
- **Cystic fibrosis**—Cystic fibrosis appears among all ethnic groups but is most common among Caucasians of Northern European descent. However, certain mutations of the cystic fibrosis gene are associated with Ashkenazi (German/Eastern European) Jews. (Because of the historically high rate of inbreeding among East-

ern European Jews, they tend to have many ethnically linked genetic conditions.) Cystic fibrosis (CF) is an inherited disease and is the most common genetic cause of infant mortality, as infants who suffer from it struggle against a thick, sticky mucus that clogs their lungs and interferes with their breathing. The disease makes it difficult for them to gain weight, and they tend to wheeze and cough. Often, the adults who suffer from cystic fibrosis are infertile; some men suffer from CF-related infertility even when they have no other symptoms of the disease. Although life expectancy has traditionally been shorter for those with CF, new treatments are fast becoming available.

- **Thalassemia**—An inherited blood disorder found among people of Asian (alpha-thalassemia) or Mediterranean (beta-thalassemia) descent, causing a disturbance in hemoglobin production. Since the gene for beta-thalassemia is carried by some 3 percent of the world's population, the American Society for Reproductive Medicine recommends that all childbearing couples be given a complete blood count (CBC) to find out whether the person has *enough* red blood cells, as well as a test of *mean corpuscle volume* (MCV) to find whether the corpuscles—red blood cells—are normal or "skinny." "Skinny" red blood cells could indicate the more common iron-deficiency anemia. The person with normal red blood cells—but too few of them—could have thalassemia. The milder form of the disease, thalassemia minor, produces only mild anemia. The more severe thalassemia major can cause serious anemia and may even be fatal.

- **Tay-Sachs disease**—This condition is most often found among Ashkenazi Jews (100 times more frequently than in the general population) and French Canadians. Caused by a problem with the way that nerve cells metabolize fat, Tay-Sachs results in progressive mental deterioration, blindness, paralysis, seizures, and death by age four. Approximately 1 in every 27 Ashkenazi Jews carries the gene for this condition.

- **Gaucher disease**—This genetic disorder causes the accumulation of fats in various places in the body, sometimes leading to an enlarged liver or spleen or to bone damage. This disease is found mainly among Ashkenazi Jews, 4 to 9 percent of whom carry a gene for the condition, affecting 1 in 2,500 Ashkenazi Jewish children. Treatment is available, but it's very expensive.

- **Canavan disease**—This fatal, inherited disease affects the body's ability to break down a key protein known as N-acetylaspartate acid (NAA). Because NAA can't be broken down, it accumulates in the brain, causing brain damage, severe mental retardation, and, about 50 percent of the time, seizures. About 1 in 38 Ashkenazi Jews carries a gene for this disease, although other ethnic groups may also get it.
- **Niemann-Pick disease**—Like the other conditions we've mentioned, this disease can be found in any ethnic group but is most common among Ashkenazi Jews. It, too, is rare and can be screened for.

Other less common disorders you may be screened for include Bloom's syndrome and Fanconi's anemia.

Family-Linked Genetic Conditions

- **Hemophilia**—This is a condition in which a person's blood does not clot properly, so that even a small injury can cause fatal bleeding. If you or the baby's father has any family history of hemophilia, you should be screened.
- **Duchenne muscular dystrophy**—This muscle-wasting disease also has a family link; usually, doctors screen only when there's a family history.
- **Huntington's chorea**—One of the few genetic diseases that appears late in life is Huntington's chorea, a painful and degenerative disease of the nervous system. Doctors usually screen for it only when there's a family history, since it tends to appear long after child-bearing age. Many people prefer not to be screened, since knowing about an unpreventable disease that may appear many years from now is an exceptional emotional strain.
- **Fragile X syndrome**—This "weak link" on the X chromosome affects 1 in 1,500 males and 1 in 2,500 females. It can result in mild to severe learning disabilities, mental retardation, or autism. If either you or your partner has a close relative who is mentally

What's in a Gene?

When the egg and sperm unite to form an embryo, the new life gets half of its genetic material from each of its parents. The embryo contains 23 pairs of chromosomes, with each parent contributing one member of each pair. The chromosomes in turn carry our *genes.*

Genes bear much of the basic information that makes us who we are—instructions for our growth patterns, biochemistry, and metabolism, as well as the basis for our hair color, eye color, and other aspects of our appearance.

Some disorders are carried through our genes as well. A child has a 1 in 2 chance of inheriting a *dominant* disorder if one parent has it.

If only one parent has a *recessive* disorder, however, then the child will not inherit the condition—although he or she may become a carrier, just as the parent was. If both parents are carrying the same recessive disorder, their child has a 1 in 4 chance of actually getting the disease.

Some genetic disorders travel only from the mother to the son, or from either parent to the daughter. (Because that type of disorder travels on the X chromosome, it's called an *X-linked inheritance.*) Baldness, for example, is passed on from mother to son.

Some genetic disorders result not from inheritance, but from problems that occurred while the fetus's chromosomes and genes were forming. These problems become more frequent as the mother—and her eggs—get older. Down's syndrome, for example, is far more likely in the children of older mothers.

retarded, slow to develop, or autistic, that relative can be tested to see if he or she suffers from Fragile X. You and your partner can also be tested to see if you are carriers.

Coping with Genetic Risks

Many of my patients become quite anxious at the thought of genetic risks—particularly if there's a family history of problems, or, alternatively, when either partner has been adopted or knows little about his or her family history.

If you're nervous about genetic problems, I'd urge you to keep some perspective. In most cases, you and your partner have a very small chance of passing on any problematic condition. And a number of interventions and tests are available after you do become pregnant.

If you and your partner are both carriers of either a recessive or a dominant gene for some conditions, you might consider the test known as CVS—*chorionic villus sampling*—in which a sample is taken from the infant's *chorion* (see Chapter 6) at about 10 to 11 weeks. Alternatively, *amniocentesis*—a sampling of the amniotic fluid—can be performed at 15 to 16 weeks. If abortion is an option for you, either of these tests gives you time to make that choice without undue risk.

Even if you elect to carry to term, knowing that one or both of your fetuses suffers from a genetic disease can help you and your doctor confront the higher risks involved in your pregnancy. The knowledge can also help ensure that the newborns will get prompt intervention to optimize their care. (For more on prenatal testing and decision-making, see Chapter 6.)

One of the most interesting cutting-edge tests available is *preimplantation genetic diagnosis,* or PGD. This relatively new procedure might be appropriate if you and/or your partner are at particularly high risk for passing on a particular genetic disease and if you're uncomfortable with the option of aborting affected fetuses.

PGD must be performed using IVF techniques, in which embryos are cultivated outside the womb and then implanted into the mother's uterus. Before implantation, a tiny amount of material is selected from each in vitro embryo and then tested, so that only those without the disease are implanted back into your uterus. Possibly, the tiny embryo might somehow be at risk from the testing itself—although so far no study has turned up any such risk. The advantage is that you can be relatively sure that you're not carrying any children affected by a particular genetic disease.

My patient Eileen had an interesting approach to this test. Huntington's chorea ran in her family, but since the disease appears late in

Who Should Consider Genetic Counseling?

Genetic counseling can help you find out more about the risks your unborn children face from genetic diseases. You may want to consider genetic counseling if:

- you're concerned about a disorder or birth defect that runs in your family, including *neural-tube defects* (such as spina bifida) and *hemophilia;*
- you think you might have an inherited disorder;
- you're worried about genetic disorders common to your ethnic group;
- you're pregnant or planning to get pregnant past age 34;
- you already have a child with mental retardation, an inherited disorder, or a birth defect;
- you've had two or more miscarriages or babies that died in infancy;
- you're having a baby with a first cousin or close blood relative.

life, she didn't yet know if she herself was affected. Eileen's mother had died of that condition, so she herself had a 1 in 2 chance of being affected—and a 1 in 4 chance of passing the disease on to her child. She was trying to conceive through IVF, and she didn't want to carry an embryo affected by the disease. But she also didn't want to find out whether she herself was affected, preferring to hope for the best rather than to know the worst.

How could she have her embryos tested without finding out more about her own condition? Certainly, the discovery of Huntington's chorea in even a single embryo would be proof positive that she herself was affected.

Finally, my patient decided to be tested "confidentially." She instructed the IVF specialists to perform PGD and to avoid transplanting any embryos affected with Huntington's. But she also told them *not* to tell her if they found any such embryos. That way, she could shield her potential children from the disease without finding out whether she had it herself.

Becoming pregnant should ideally be one of the most joyful experiences of your life. There will be much about pregnancy, childbirth, and the raising of your children that you will *not* be able to anticipate or prepare for. So plan for what you can! The more planning you can do ahead of time, the more you will be able to relax and enjoy the ride.

3.

The Biology of Multiple Pregnancy

B efore you had a more personal reason to be interested in twins, you may have thought there were only two types: *fraternal,* or the kind that don't necessarily look alike, and *identical,* the kind that supposedly *do* look alike.

In fact, there are several different types of twins—and many biological variations among other multiples as well. Moreover, the common terms *fraternal* and *identical* are fairly misleading—"fraternal" twins can include two sisters or a brother–sister pair, while "identical" twins do not necessarily resemble each other in every way (though they *do* tend to look alike).

Determining what kind of twins you've got is probably one of the first things your doctor will want to do. This information will help him or her decide what type of monitoring you should have, what hazards to look out for, and what kind of delivery you're likely to have.

Meanwhile, knowing more about the biology of twinning can help you and your partner visualize what's going on inside your body. So even if you avoided your high-school biology class like the plague, get ready for a quick biology lesson now. Given your new personal interest in the topic, it may be even a subject you enjoy!

Fertilization: Where It All Begins

Let's start with the basics: how babies are made. By the time you reach puberty, your ovaries contain a number of eggs, one of which is released during every regular menstrual cycle in a process known as *ovulation*. If you've had ART, your doctor may have stimulated this process with some kind of medication, a process known as *ovulation induction*. Usually, the ovaries release only a single egg each month, but sometimes—through natural causes or because of the extra stimulation of ART—more than one egg is released.

For the moment, let's follow the path of just a single egg as it travels through the Fallopian tube to the uterus (womb). When you have unprotected sexual intercourse, millions of sperm make their way up the Fallopian tube, where one of them may intercept the egg. If one sperm reaches the egg in time (before or during ovulation, while the egg is still in the outer third of the tube) and penetrates it successfully, the egg is *fertilized,* and the mother's and father's cells unite to form a new entity. (See Figure 1.)

The cells of the fertilized egg continue to grow and divide as the egg moves up into the uterus, looking for a hospitable spot on the uterine wall. An unfertilized egg does *not* implant itself into the wall and is shed with the uterine lining during menstruation. A fertilized egg, however, attaches itself to the uterus and begins to grow.

Monozygotic or "Identical" Twins

The fertilization process up to this point is pretty much the same for both singletons and monozygotic twins. *Monozygotic* means *from one zygote,* which is the term that describes the initial fertilized egg. A monozygotic pair of twins comes from a single egg fertilized by a single sperm. This zygote contains 46 chromosomes—the bearers of genetic information—half from the mother's egg, half from the father's sperm. (That's why your child has a 1 in 2 chance of inheriting your characteristics and a similar chance of inheriting those of the father.) (See Figure 2.)

In monozygotic twinning, however, the chromosomes double in

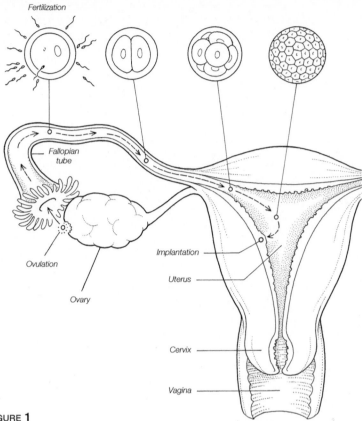

Fertilization

Fallopian
tube

Ovulation

Ovary

Implantation

Uterus

Cervix

Vagina

FIGURE 1

number, and the fertilized egg splits in two. We don't fully know why this happens, though it seems to have to do with a delay either in the zygote's growth process or in the time it takes to implant itself into the uterus. The age of the ovum may also be involved.

What we do know is that monozygotic twins start out with identical genetic material. That's why this type of twin is considered identical, even though the twins generally develop different likes, dislikes, abilities, and personalities. They may also develop distinctive appearances, including different heights and weights.

However, monozygotic twins are always the same sex, and they do begin life with similar hair and eye colors, blood groups, body scents, dental impressions, and other distinguishing characteristics. Their electroencephalograms (measurements of the electrical activity in the brain) are likewise similar, as are their cardiovascular measurements (information about their hearts and circulatory systems).

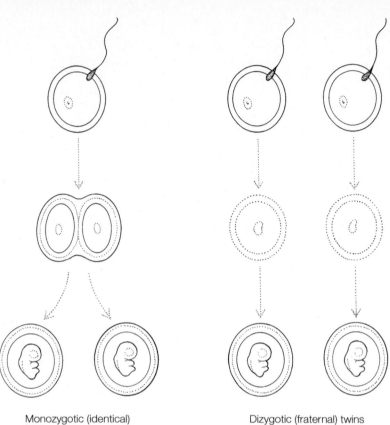

Monozygotic (identical)
twins occur when one egg
is fertilized by one sperm.

Dizygotic (fraternal) twins
occur when two eggs are
fertilized by two sperm.

FIGURE 2

Monozygotic twins may also have similar tendencies toward the same types of disorders, such as asthma, diabetes, depression, schizophrenia, and cancer, although one twin may be more severely affected than the other. A monozygotic twin could also be an organ donor for the other twin, with no need for the antirejection therapy usually required for donations.

Some 3.5 to 4 births in 1,000 are monozygotic twins, a rate that seems to be fairly constant throughout the world. However, for reasons that we don't fully understand, women who are having ART seem to conceive monozygotic twins at a rate two to three times higher than in unassisted pregnancies. Also, if you are a monozygotic twin, you seem to have a higher chance of having same-sex twins of your own.

About one-third of all twins are monozygotic, and of these, half are male and the other half are female. About one-fourth of all monozygotic twins are known as "mirror twins" because they are mirror images of each other. That is, a birthmark that appears on one twin's left side may appear on the other twin's right. In rare cases, even an organ such as the appendix may appear in mirror formation. One mirror twin is likely to be left-handed, while the other is right-handed, and they tend to cross thumbs, arms, and legs in opposite directions.

Generally, multiple pregnancies run a higher risk of birth defects, with monozygotic twins facing a risk that is 2.5 times as great as for dizygotic twins.

Dizygotic or "Fraternal" Twins

Dizygotic twinning accounts for about two-thirds of all twins. The rate of dizygotic twins seems to vary by population, with the highest rates occurring among Africans who live in Africa, the lowest rates among Asians who live in Asia, and rates in between occurring among Europeans or North Americans of European descent. People of Asian ancestry living outside of Asia seem to have higher rates of twinning than Asians living in Asia. Some studies also suggest that your chance of having dizygotic twins is increased if you yourself are a dizygotic twin.

To produce dizygotic twins, two eggs are fertilized by two different sperm. The two eggs may be from the same ovary, or each may be from a different ovary. Likewise, the two eggs may be fertilized on the same occasion or, rarely, on two separate occasions, up to a week or so apart.

An interesting but extremely rare type of dizygotic twinning results from *superfetation,* in which a second egg is fertilized in a second reproductive cycle. In theory, a woman could experience superfetation any time during the first three months of a pregnancy, but the hormonal changes of pregnancy make this unlikely. Likewise, it's theoretically possible for the twins to have separate birth dates—days or even months apart—but instances of this are exceedingly rare, as are cases of women conceiving twins with two different fathers. (See Figure 3.)

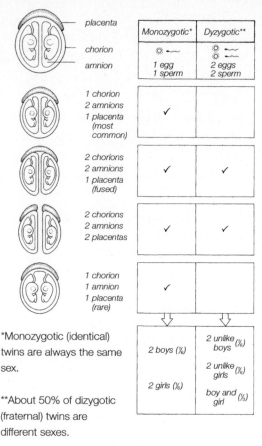

	Monozygotic*	Dyzygotic**
placenta / chorion / amnion	1 egg / 1 sperm	2 eggs / 2 sperm
1 chorion / 2 amnions / 1 placenta (most common)	✓	
2 chorions / 2 amnions / 1 placenta (fused)	✓	✓
2 chorions / 2 amnions / 2 placentas	✓	✓
1 chorion / 1 amnion / 1 placenta (rare)	✓	
	2 boys (⅓) / 2 girls (⅓)	2 unlike boys (⅓) / 2 unlike girls (⅓) / boy and girl (⅓)

*Monozygotic (identical) twins are always the same sex.

**About 50% of dizygotic (fraternal) twins are different sexes.

FIGURE 3

About half of all dizygotic twins are same-sex pairs, and half are male–female.

Dizygotic twins run a risk of chromosomal abnormalities that is almost twice as high as that of singletons, but no higher risk of nonchromosomal structural problems.

Higher-Order Multiples

If you're pregnant with triplets, quads, or higher-order multiples, you may have undergone monozygotic twinning, multizygotic twinning, or some combination of the two. The famous Dionne quintuplets were monozygotic, for example, with a single egg splitting into five parts. On the other hand, ART is making dizygotic reproduction more common than ever, as many forms of ART increase the number of eggs available to be fertilized. A combination of in vitro fertilization (IVF) and embryo transfer, in which several eggs are fertilized outside the mother's body and then transferred back into the womb, vastly increases the chances of dizygotic or multizygotic reproduction, with two or more eggs growing separately, first outside, then inside, the mother's body.

At the same time, for reasons we don't yet understand, IVF also seems to produce a higher-than-average incidence of monozygotic twins. As fertility treatments become ever more widespread, we continue to learn more about their relationship to multiple births.

Monozygotic triplets may also occur, although this is the least common type. More often, triplets are the result of three separately fertilized eggs (trizygotic triplets). Alternatively, one pair of monozygotic twins and a second fertilized egg might result in triplets. With a higher number of fetuses, either or both processes might be involved; thus quadruplets, for example, could arise from one, two, three, or four ova!

The Development of the Placenta

So far, we've taken the story of conception and pregnancy through its first week. That's how long it takes for the fertilized egg to reach the uterus and for the *placenta* to begin to grow.

Let's start by seeing how the placenta functions in a singleton pregnancy. The placenta is a sac that nourishes the growing fetus. It's mostly made up of the mother's tissue, though some fetal tissue is also involved. By the time the baby is ready to be born, the placenta will be at least six inches in diameter and about two inches thick.

The placenta houses tiny projections called *villi,* which cover a huge surface area totaling 150 square feet. Inside the villi are the fetal blood vessels, which, if linked, would extend for over 30 miles.

The mother and fetus each has his/her own separate circulatory system—that's how babies can have different blood types than their parents—but nutrients and waste products are exchanged through the villi, which are constantly bathed by the mother's blood.

Amnions and Chorions

Let's continue to look at a typical singleton pregnancy. Within the placenta, the single fetus is contained in a sac consisting of two membranes growing out of the placenta's edge. This sac is filled with amniotic fluid, so called because the inner membrane is known as the *amnion*. The amnion is clear and shiny, with no blood vessels, and it can easily be detached from the placenta.

The outer membrane is called the *chorion*. It is relatively opaque, in part because it does contain blood vessels. A ridge running along the underside of the placenta shows where the chorion is attached.

The membranous sac formed by the amnion and chorion contains a protective fluid that acts as a shock absorber, helps maintain an even temperature, and gives the fetus room to grow and move freely. (See Figure 4.)

As you might expect, different types of twins have different ways of sharing placentas, amnions, and chorions, depending on when the twinning occurs. The later the twinning takes place, the more likely the twins are to share an amnion or a chorion. That's because chorions form at about Day 4, so if the division takes place later than that, the twins will develop within the same chorion. Likewise, since amnions form at about Day 8, twins who develop later than that will live within the same amnion, though this situation is far less common.

Monozygotic twins formed by an egg splitting at later than 13½ days may not represent full duplication of all the embryonic material, with the result that twins may be incomplete or malformed in some way. For example, such twins may be *conjoined,* sharing one or more organs (occurring in 1 in 500 twin pregnancies or 1 in 50,000 to 80,000 deliveries). (For more on conjoined twins and other twin structural problems, see Chapter 13.)

Thus it is possible to talk about:

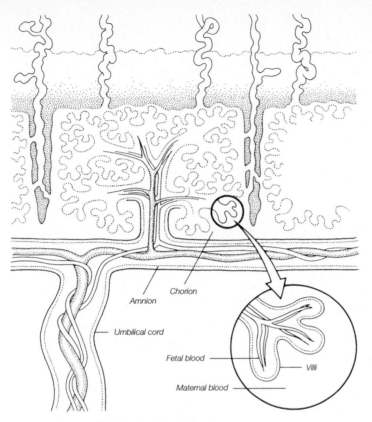

FIGURE 4. A look inside the placenta.

- *monoamniotic twins*—who share an amnion (and therefore also a chorion);
- *monochorionic twins*—who each have their own amnion within a shared chorion;
- *dichorionic twins*—who have separate amnions and separate chorions.

There are four possibilities for monozygotic twins:

- *1 chorion, 1 amnion, 1 placenta*—the most rare;
- *1 chorion, 2 amnions, 1 placenta*—the most common;
- *2 chorions, 2 amnions, fused placentas;*
- *2 chorions, 2 amnions, 2 separate placentas.*

Because dizygotic twins develop earlier, they are always dichorionic and diamniotic. That is, the body, recognizing that there are two

HOW MONOZYGOTIC TWINS DEVELOP

Monozygotic twinning—takes place when a fertilized ovum divides, sometime between Day 2 and Day 17 after fertilization.

....

Dichorionic–diamniotic twinning—takes place when the division occurs within 72 hours of twinning; accounts for some 30 percent of all monozygotic twins.

....

Monochorionic–diamniotic twinning—takes place when ovum divides between 4 and 8 days; accounts for some 68 percent of all monozygotic twins.

....

Monochorionic–monoamniotic twinning—takes place when ovum divides between 8 and 13½ days after fertilization; accounts for 1–2 percent of all monozygotic twins.

babies growing within it, provides each with its own separate amniotic sac covered by its own chorion. However, dizygotic twins may have either separate or fused placentas. (See Figure 5.)

Monoamniotic Twins

Of all monozygotic twins, only 1 to 2 percent are monoamniotic. This is fortunate, as the greatest risk of complication is associated with these twins. (As you can imagine, sharing a sac increases the risk of the twins being entangled and other complications, while sharing amniotic fluid means that whatever happens to one twin is extremely likely to affect the other.) This type of twinning may be marked by such anomalies as only one artery in the umbilical cord, rather than two, or insertion of the cord into the membranes, rather than into the placenta. Monoamniotic twins also face the risk of cord entanglement.

Monochorionic Twins

Some 68 percent of all monozygotic twins share a chorion while having their own separate amnions. Monochorionic twins by defi-

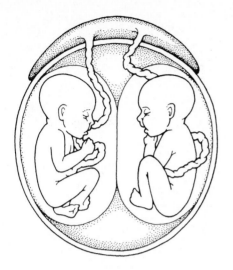

Monochorionic
Diamniotic
(Monozygotic Twins)

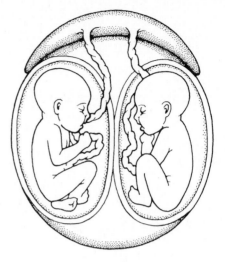

Dichorionic
Diamniotic
(Monozygotic or Dizygotic Twins)

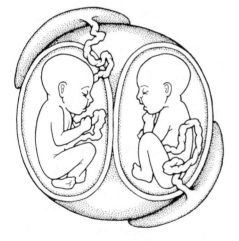

Dichorionic
Diamniotic
(Monozygotic or Dizygotic Twins)

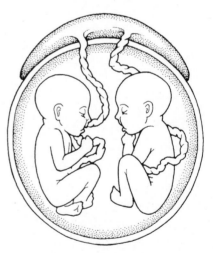

Monochorionic
Monoamniotic
(Monozygotic Twins—very rare)

FIGURE 5

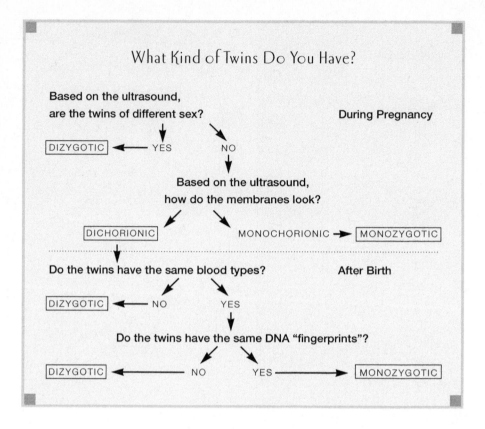

What Kind of Twins Do You Have?

Based on the ultrasound, are the twins of different sex?   During Pregnancy

DIZYGOTIC ← YES   NO

Based on the ultrasound, how do the membranes look?

DICHORIONIC   MONOCHORIONIC → MONOZYGOTIC

Do the twins have the same blood types?   After Birth

DIZYGOTIC ← NO   YES

Do the twins have the same DNA "fingerprints"?

DIZYGOTIC ← NO   YES → MONOZYGOTIC

nition share a single placenta. Although there are fewer risks and complications with monochorionic–diamniotic twins than with monoamniotic twins, this type of twinning still contributes to a higher-risk pregnancy, with greater chances of fetal anomalies and such complications as twin–twin transfusion. (For more on this type of complication, see Chapter 13.)

Dichorionic Twins

As we've seen, all dizygotic twins fall into this category—each has its own separate inner and outer membrane as well as its own placenta. About 25 percent of all monozygotic twins also fall within this category.

How Do You Know?

As you can see, there are lots of reasons why you'll want to know whether your twins are "identical" or "fraternal"—that is, monozygotic or dizygotic. In many cases, your doctor will be able to figure this out before birth, but if not, he or she can determine your babies' zygosity soon after delivery.

To figure out this important question, your doctor will ask a number of different questions, beginning with his or her initial diagnosis of twins.

Here's one more way of looking at it:

- All dizygotic twins are dichorionic.
- Not all dichorionic twins are dizygotic.
- Monozygotic twins can be either monochorionic or dichorionic.
- All monochorionic twins are monozygotic.

4.

How Do You Feel?: Psychological Issues

❧

"What do you *mean* I'm going to have twins?" my patient Miriam said when I gave her the news. Her husband, Ira, was supposed to have come with her for their first ultrasound, but he'd gotten held up with a client at his busy law practice. Miriam herself had taken time off from the department store where she was a buyer, but she'd been looking impatiently at her watch for quite a while, worried about being on time for her noon meeting. Now she was staring at me in disbelief. "It was already enough of a challenge for us to manage *one* baby!" she told me. "How in the *world* will we ever manage two?"

Natalie's reaction was just the opposite—she looked at me as though I'd just given her the most wonderful present in the world. "Wow," she sighed. "All my life I dreamed of having twins. But I never thought it would actually happen. I can't believe it's happening to me."

Over the years I've been in practice, I've seen an entire spectrum of reactions to twins, from shock and dismay to joy and gratitude—not to mention the parents who run the entire gamut of emotions all by themselves! Any pregnancy is a major life change, but a multiple pregnancy is an even more dramatic transformation. In this chapter, I'll help you sort through some of the issues you may be coping with as you come to terms with the news of your upcoming twins, triplets, or quads. I'll also suggest some approaches that may help you to feel more relaxed, secure, and in touch with your body.

The Mind–Body Connection

Although there's no hard medical evidence linking state of mind and health of body, I've seen time and time again that women who are more relaxed and positive tend to do better than women who are overwhelmed with household problems, stresses at work, and anxiety over their pregnancy. The more you can relax and enjoy this unique time in your life, the more easily your body can adjust to all the new demands.

Let's be very clear about this: I'm *not* suggesting that if you're feeling overwhelmed or stressed out it's "your fault" or you are somehow to blame for fatigue, discomfort, or any complications that may accompany your pregnancy. I *am* suggesting that you take your emotional life as seriously as you take your physical health and that you recognize how emotionally and physically demanding a multiple pregnancy is. That may mean taking time off from work or making clear to your boss and coworkers that you will be doing less for a time. It may mean reaching out to friends and relatives for increased help with child care and the household. And it may mean renegotiating responsibilities with your partner, as well as asking for various kinds of emotional and practical support—a massage, the chance to luxuriate in a warm bath, some quiet time at the end of the day to rest and recoup.

In this spirit, I'd like to repeat a message I'll be promoting throughout this book: A multiple pregnancy poses higher risks and more demands than a single pregnancy, and women who are pregnant with twins, triplets, and quads should be prepared to make more changes in their lives than women who are pregnant with singletons. Your pregnant sister may regale the family with stories of how she cooked Thanksgiving dinner for twenty during her ninth month, while you, in your third month, can barely boil water for tea. Your pregnant coworker might have stayed up half the night on a crucial presentation the day before delivery, while you find yourself nodding out at 3:00 P.M. every afternoon. And your partner may remember how during your previous pregnancies you happily did your half of the laundry, the shopping, and the cooking—while *this* time, you might think it's a good day if you manage to clear away the breakfast dishes before the sun goes down.

Some women adjust to the greater changes in their bodies without great difficulty, while others are encumbered with the heavier weight, increased pressure, and greater discomfort that challenge multiple moms. Of course, you're going to need more medical attention than singleton moms—as you can see from the rest of this book! But you might allow yourself more time to adjust emotionally as well.

Common Fears and Concerns: "How Will I Ever Take Care of *So Many* Babies?!"

If you've undergone Assisted Reproductive Technology (ART) or in vitro fertilization (IVF), you may be prepared for the possibility of a multiple pregnancy. But to many multiple moms—and their partners—the news comes as a shock. Depending on your age, your financial situation, and the number of other children you have, the initial discovery can feel overwhelming.

I remember when I first realized I was having twins. It was my second pregnancy, and I felt that my uterine size was greater than it should be. A colleague admonished me: "Don't be your own doctor!" Of course, my sonogram confirmed my suspicion—it *was* twins! I have learned this lesson so many times from the other side of the examining table—the need to respect the patient's opinion. As both doctor and patient, I've seen that doctors don't listen to their patients enough, whereas asking the patient how she feels and what she's thinking turns out to be an amazingly rich source of information time and again.

When I discovered my multiple pregnancy, so many thoughts raced through my mind—joy at the thought of producing *two* siblings for my three-year-old to play with; happiness that I had found an "efficient" way of producing more children per pregnancy, especially given my schedule; a lot of fears about balancing my career and family life and about the risks of premature labor and birth. What most helped me get through this challenging time was taking it all one day at a time—a philosophy that continues to serve me well as mother of four and doctor to other pregnant women.

One day at a time was a philosophy that Miriam also came to embrace. "That first day in your office," she told me recently, "I thought my world had come to an end. Of *course* I was thrilled that our babies were healthy, normal, and all the rest of it—but come on! I had *twins*! All I could think was, oh, God, *two* night feedings, *two* sets of infants crying on different shifts, *two* college funds to pay into. Ira and I had been so excited when we found out I was pregnant—and now we had to cope with *this*?"

Sarah, on the other hand, was 39. She and her partner had accepted that they would probably be able to have only one child, even though both had come from big families and were close to their brothers and sisters. "So when you told me I had triplets," Sarah recalled, "I just thought, 'Great! Instant family!' Worry about the complications didn't hit home till later."

Whether your first reaction is dread or delight, you and your partner will probably find yourselves having a whole range of feelings, including hope, excitement, fear, anxiety, and a preoccupation with practical concerns. Here are some of the most common concerns I've noticed:

- I'm too old to take care of so many kids—I won't have the energy!
- What kinds of risks am I facing?
- Will I make it through the delivery?
- Do I have to have a C-section?
- *Can* I have a C-section?
- Can I deliver naturally, or will I have to have drugs?
- *Can* I have drugs, or will they hurt the babies?
- Will *all* my babies be all right?
- Will I have to stop work?
- Will I have to stay in bed?
- When can I go back to work?
- I wanted one child—not two (or three, or four)! I just didn't bargain for this!

- I'll be okay—but my husband/partner won't. I feel like I've tricked him/her somehow.
- How will we get any sleep ever again?
- Will they be crying *all* the time?
- Oh, my God, I'll be big as a house!
- My older children will be so embarrassed—I'll look *so* pregnant.
- I don't know anyone else who has multiples—who's going to help me through this?
- Where will I ever find a sitter?
- How can we afford two (or three or four) of everything?
- Am I supposed to dress them all alike? How will they ever develop their own personalities?
- How will I tell them apart?
- I don't have enough to give *two* (or three or four) babies—I'm afraid they'll be shortchanged.
- How will the grandparents react? Will they have favorites?
- Taking care of my other children was going to be hard enough with *one* new baby—but with *two* (or three or four) it's just impossible!

Common Hopes and Fantasies: "I'll Feel Like Supermom!"

Besides the fears and concerns, there are the hopes and fantasies. Here are some of the ones I've encountered, in myself and in my patients:

- Wow! Two (or three or four) at once! I'll feel like Supermom— the original earth mother!
- Great! Instant family!
- Hey—efficiency is my middle name!
- After all these years of trying to get pregnant, getting *two* (or three or four) babies at once feels like a special blessing.
- Good—they can play with each other and keep each other company.
- I've heard they actually cry *less*. They don't get lonely when they wake up, so they cry only when they're hungry, not when they need company.

- It's so special to have a twin. Each of my babies will always have a brother or sister to be very, very close to.
- Right from the beginning, they're going to learn to be very good at sharing.
- There's something kind of magical about twins (and triplets, and quads). It will be fascinating to watch how similar they look—and yet how different they are.
- This way, my partner and I will both be very involved. There will be one for him (or her) and one for me!
- I didn't want to get pregnant twice, or to stretch out the years I'm taking care of young children—but I never liked the idea of having an only child. This way, I get to have my cake and eat it too.

Coping with Your Feelings: "What Do We Do Now?"

You may have some, all, or none of these feelings—or you may have other fears, concerns, and fantasies that I haven't mentioned. Either way, take heart. It's normal for you and your partner to have a whole range of feelings about any pregnancy. A multiple pregnancy *is* more demanding, and also less familiar—you've probably watched lots of friends and relatives go through a singleton pregnancy and early child rearing, but you may never ever have known anyone who had twins, triplets, or quads (although they are becoming more common every year).

The important thing is to be aware of your feelings and to not judge yourself—or your partner. Give yourselves time and talk about the feelings as they come up—with your partner, a relative, or a non-judgmental friend. You might also find it helpful to write down how you feel in a private journal, where you can acknowledge all the different reactions you've had, including the ones you're not so proud of. (*I hate the thought of getting so* fat! *I think Joe can be a good father to* one *child, but I'm not sure he's got it in him to take care of two at once. I'm a pretty selfish person. I just don't think I'll be able to give enough of myself to* three *babies.*)

Then, when the smoke has cleared, start to separate the fantasies and nightmares from more realistic concerns. Remember that all of your feelings are valid *as feelings,* but they don't all equally reflect reality. You may face some additional risks—but find out more from your doctor before you let your fears run away with you. Yes, you may have to spend more time away from your job than with a singleton pregnancy—but you may find that your boss and your coworkers are happy to cooperate. Child care is a tough issue for virtually all parents, but maybe you can tap into some as-yet-undiscovered resources—foreign college students looking for live-in au pair situations, another pregnant mom who wants to switch off child care, local high-school students who can tutor your third-grader with his homework. It might help you to make two lists: *Fears* and *Realistic Concerns.* Give yourself the space to have your fears and address them, while turning to the realistic concerns in a more practical spirit.

Support Groups: "So It's *Not* Just Me!"

One of the best things you can do for yourself—and perhaps for your partner as well—is to get into a multiple parents' support group. These vary from an informal network of mothers who met by chance at the park to multigenerational parents' clubs associated with a local church, synagogue, or community center. Parents of multiples *do* face special problems, and it helps to know that the various physical, emotional, financial, and social issues you encounter aren't unique to you or your family.

"Honestly, my support group saved my life," Sarah says. "After the first wave of euphoria wore off, I realized that I'd never even known anyone who had triplets. I had the feeling that my mother was kind of intimidated by the whole thing, and my two sisters were all for giving me advice—but their experiences were so different. I had morning sickness right away, for example, and it didn't let up for several months—that was nothing like what happened to them. Luckily, I'd found a group before the end of my first trimester, so when the morning sickness went on into the fourth month, I had two other pregnant women telling me that they'd been through that the month before."

Miriam, on the other hand, said she "wasn't the type" to talk about her problems "with a group of strangers."

"I don't want to insult anyone," she says, "but to me, support groups just seem like a waste of time. When I was pregnant, I had only a few spare minutes each day—and it's even worse now that the twins are here. I don't want to waste that precious time listening to women yak about their problems."

Obviously, the decision to find a support group is a very individual choice! But if you'd like to check out a group, take a look at the Resources section of this book, where we've listed some national organizations that may have local chapters. Or you might try one of these other ideas to locate the support group that is right for you:

- Search the Internet for *twins, triplets, quads,* or *multiple pregnancy.*
- Check out churches, synagogues, and other religious organizations.
- Explore various Y's, Jewish Community Centers, Parent–Teacher Associations, and other community groups.
- Ask your doctor.
- Drop by the park or playground, keep an eye out for double or triple strollers, and talk to the multiple parents you meet.

Working with Your Partner and Your Family: "Honey, I Need a Break!"

Any pregnancy brings adjustments and new demands to your partner and your other children, if you have any. Your multiple pregnancy requires even more help and cooperation from your partner, particularly if you have to spend all or part of your pregnancy in bed. (For more on bed rest, see Chapter 9.) So how do the two of you face these new challenges? Here are a few suggestions:

- **Keep each other posted.** This sounds obvious, but it can be harder than it sounds. In a busy marriage, especially if both of you are working, and most especially if you also have young children, one thing that easily gets lost is time for the two adults to talk. You and your partner will have more trouble supporting each other if you don't even know what the other wants. And your partner is likely to be far more helpful if *you've* been open and vulnerable in sharing your own feelings, fears, and concerns. "Actually, in some ways, having twins was good for our marriage," Miriam told me. "With just one baby, Ira and I might have continued on automatic pilot. With two kids, though, we really had to make time for each other, right from the start."

- **Stay in touch with yourself.** How can you communicate with your partner if *you* don't know how you feel? The normal ups and downs of pregnancy—the hormone swings, surges of energy and exhaustion, hopes and fears about the future—are likely to be intensified by a multiple pregnancy. If this is your first time around, the whole experience is likely to feel strange and at least a little confusing. If you've given birth before, you may be thrown by the differences you encounter. "My twins were my third and fourth children," explains 34-year-old Zoe. "But I'd had my first two children in my mid-twenties, and they were both singletons. I just wasn't prepared for how exhausted I'd be this time around."

- **Reach out.** If ever there was a time for an extended family, for close friends, for community support, that time is now. Figuring out how to enlist support in our individualistic, "I can do it myself" society may not be easy, especially at a time when the superachieving pregnant woman is almost a media cliché. But try to be open to a wide range of options, to let people see your needy as well as your self-reliant side, and to celebrate the many different ways that people can participate in your family life. "I've always hated to ask for help," Miriam admits. "But there was something about being pregnant with twins—it was such a dramatic situation. For the first time in my life, I felt like I had a *good* excuse for not being able to do it all myself."

Sex and Sexuality: "Where Are My Limits?"

There are two equally important aspects to sex during pregnancy: 1) what's medically advisable; 2) how you feel.

The medical part is fairly easy. In most cases, you should be able to have intercourse throughout your pregnancy. During your first trimester, your breasts may be unusually tender, so you and your part-ner may want to take this into account. If you're urinating more fre-quently, you might want to be sure to empty your bladder before intercourse. As you get bigger, having another person on top might be uncomfortable, so you may want to experiment with some other po-sitions. After the birth, your vagina may be drier, so you might need longer foreplay before you're fully lubricated. Some women like to use a water-soluble lubricant, such as K–Y jelly or Astroglide.

All other things being equal, here are a few other medical don't's:

- Your partner may like to blow air into your vagina during sex. This is perfectly safe when you're not pregnant, but during preg-nancy it could lead to a possibly fatal embolism (air bubble) in your lung.
- If something causes you to feel cramping, pain, or discomfort, don't do it.

Sometimes, of course, all other things are *not* equal. Your doctor will advise you of the times when either sexual activity in general or intercourse in particular is not advisable, such as if:

- your cervix is undergoing certain types of changes;
- your fetal membranes are ruptured;
- you're bleeding;
- you've been having preterm labor or have a history of preterm labor in other pregnancies;
- you've got a *cerclage* (a stitch holding your cervix closed, used to prevent preterm labor);
- you've been advised to undergo bed rest to prevent preterm labor.

All right, those are the medical issues. But what about the emo-tional issues?

The experience of sexuality during pregnancy is as individual as each woman who becomes pregnant. Many women feel no change in their sexual desires, while others feel decreased desire, and still others feel sexier than ever. "Those first few months were like a second hon-eymoon," recalls Natalie, while Zoe says, "Sex? Are you kidding? I was too tired to brush my teeth!"

If you or your partner associates pregnancy with being unattrac-tive, asexual, or gross, it may be difficult for one or both of you to feel sexual desire. Like Zoe, many women feel increasingly tired during pregnancy, especially a multiple pregnancy, which makes them feel less interested in sex and more interested in sleep. If your partner is doing double duty because of the pregnancy, he or she may feel tired and less sexual too. If either or both of you feel scared of the pregnancy, the delivery, or the prospect of parenthood, that can turn you off, at least temporarily. And since people associate pregnancy with motherhood, you or your partner may have conflicting feelings about a *mother* hav-ing sex.

Many women feel less sexual during pregnancy even as they desire more physical contact—being cuddled, held, massaged, or kissed. Part-ners often don't understand a pregnant woman's changing needs, and they may experience these ups and downs as a sexual rejection.

On the other hand, many couples feel a new sense of sexual free-dom during pregnancy. Before they got pregnant, they may have been preoccupied either with preventing pregnancy or with trying to con-ceive. With pregnancy, the old pressures around preventing or encour-aging conception are over, and estrogen levels are up. In this new emotional and physical environment, sexual desire may flourish. The pregnant woman may find that her libido has increased, that she's more lubricated, more sensitive, and generally more open to sensual pleasure. And some couples feel especially close as they look forward to the pregnancy, a closeness that can heighten sexual desire.

Sarah told me that pregnancy was a time when she felt comfort-able with her body for the first time in her life. "I finally didn't feel like I was supposed to be dieting," she confessed. "I would look at my big, beautiful body and think, 'This is what my body is *supposed* to do.' " Her new sense of bodily comfort made her feel both more sen-sual and more sexual.

Once again, it's clichéd but true: Self-knowledge and communica-tion are key. Knowing what you and your partner want and finding comfortable ways to talk about it are especially important if one of you feels sexual and the other doesn't, or if you both feel sexy but aren't allowed some of the positions or activities that you're used to.

Caring for the Children You Already Have: "Why Can't You Play with Us, Mommy?"

Your children will be affected by your multiple pregnancy differently, depending on how old they are. A toddler will need lots of love and attention, since he or she won't have the capacity to understand what pregnancy is or that more babies will be joining the household "in a few months." Before the age of five, children are still pretty much learning the difference between "right now" and "in a minute." They can just about grasp "wait till bedtime" or "not until tomorrow," but any time frame longer than that is beyond their reach. What young children will understand is that Mommy is suddenly too tired, too sick, or too big to do what she used to—and they won't quite know whether that's their fault or not.

As a result, many of my patients wonder about when they should tell their other children about the pregnancy. Since older children can understand more about the time involved in pregnancy, you might want to bring them in on the process earlier, especially if you're experiencing morning sickness or fatigue or any of the other symptoms of a multiple pregnancy (see Chapter 10).

Toddlers, on the other hand, don't really understand what "nine months" means, and they may worry unduly about what's going to happen to Mommy or about how those new babies are going to affect *their* lives. You might want to tell them as the second trimester ends.

I have two other suggestions for helping to ease the transition for your young children: 1) Figure out a special ritual that you and your child always share, no matter what—a special song at bedtime, a morning wake-up cuddle, or a private five minutes when he or she comes home from day care. Use this "just us" time to remind your child that no matter who else is in your life, he or she will always have a special, separate place in your heart. 2) Both during pregnancy and after the babies come, enlist the help of as many other adults as you can to give your older child the love and attention that you may not have time to provide. This is the time to ask that special aunt or uncle to commit to a weekly or monthly Saturday morning treat, or to ask Grandma, Grandpa, or your best friend to drop by for family dinners that include some private time with their "favorite." Having brothers and sisters *does* mean learning to share and compromise, but it doesn't have to mean never feeling special.

Older children will have their own issues. They *will* be able to understand that babies are coming "in a few months"—but they may be worried about how these new babies will affect *their* lives. Try to find time when they can ask their own questions and voice their own concerns.

"Sean was really furious with me, especially when he understood that there would be *two* new babies," Zoe recalls. "He was eight when I had the twins, but he had been the baby, and I think he was just scared that no one would have time for him anymore, especially when he saw how soon I couldn't do certain things with him and how busy Nick was buying all the baby furniture and other stuff. Lissa was thrilled—she was nine, just at the age when it seems like fun to play mother. But Sean and I really had to keep talking things through."

Preteens and teenagers may see your very visible pregnancy as an unwelcome reminder that you are a sexual person. As they struggle with their own sexual identities, they may feel embarrassed about this public sign of yours. There's not much you can do about this, except give them the space to talk about their feelings and try not to take anything personally.

One thing that many families with children ages five and up find helpful is a "family council." This is a family meeting that can occur on a regular basis—say, every Sunday evening—or whenever someone in the family wants to call a meeting. All family members must attend and agree to talk honestly about their feelings. Often children who are anxious about the arrival of new family members feel reassured that there is an "official" place for them in the family structure.

"When we had our first family meeting, Sean started in with his usual list of complaints—there wouldn't be any time for him, the babies would ruin all his stuff—all the things we'd been talking about for days," Zoe remembers. "Then Nick said, 'Okay, Sean, that's the problem. What are your ideas for the solution?' He was absolutely floored—

but then he started making suggestions. I really think that was when things started to turn around for him."

Coping with Community Reactions: "Aren't You Pretty Far Along by Now?"

If you've been pregnant before, you already know: Pregnancy is a very *public* condition. For some reason, perfect strangers who would never dare comment on your clothes or your hairstyle feel free to comment on your size, shape, and probable due date. The bigger you get, the more comments you attract, so if you're pregnant with twins, triplets, or quads, get ready for a *lot* of comments. You'll also find that lots of people will be asking to touch your stomach—or even reaching out and patting it without permission!

I've never been sure of the best way to handle this kind of public response, and of course, *your* reactions will vary depending on your personality, your mood, and how much sleep you got last night. The good part, of course, is that people can come through for you in wonderful ways, offering you seats on public transportation and allowing you to move to the front of long lines at the bakery. Since you really *shouldn't* be on your feet for long periods of time (again, see Chapter 9), take all the help you can get—and if the offers don't come, don't be afraid to ask! This is one time when looking more pregnant than you are pays off.

Just for You: Self-Nurture and Self-Care

Throughout this chapter, we've talked a lot about negotiating with others. Here are some things that you can do "just for you"—ways to help yourself relax and embrace the changes in your body, your feelings, and your life. Maybe only one of these ideas will appeal to you; maybe you'll like a few; maybe every one will sound good. Either way, let your instincts be your guide. And whether these suggestions work for you or not, find your own ways to pamper, care for, and listen to yourself. In the end, only you know exactly what your pregnancy is like—and what you need to make it through.

- **Relaxation techniques.** These vary widely. Some people like to make tapes for themselves, telling themselves to relax first their toes, then their ankles, then their shins, and so on, right on up to the crown of the skull. (It seems to work better to relax up instead of down.) Other people like to buy relaxation tapes, either white noise, sounds of nature, or tapes on which other people instruct you to relax or to meditate on soothing images. Still other people like to simply relax—to find a block of time from ten minutes to half an hour, sit or lie in a comfortable position, and allow themselves to become aware of their own bodies, breathing deeply. Music, incense, candles, a warm bath, or some combination thereof can all add to the relaxation. I recommend finding this kind of quiet time at least once a day. You'll be amazed at how much it refreshes you and how much more gracefully and efficiently you handle the rest of your day's duties.

- **Self-hypnosis.** This is a technique that extends relaxation an extra step. Some people use it simply to relax; others rely on it to address physical or emotional complaints, such as headache, upset stomach, asthma, anxiety, and sleep disturbances. Basically, self-hypnosis is a way of putting yourself into a hypnotic trance—a deeply relaxed state in which you are highly suggestible—and using that state to help you heal various symptoms. (People also use self-hypnosis to quit smoking and to ease caffeine withdrawal.) If this approach to your body interests you, get a referral to a hypnotist from a psychotherapist or counseling center. A hypnotist can teach you how to practice self-hypnosis, which you can then use to address the various discomforts of a multiple pregnancy.

- **Visualization.** Visualization is related to self-hypnosis, but it doesn't require being in a hypnotic trance, merely in a relaxed state. It involves visualizing your body both as it is and as you would like it to be. Many people feel comforted by imagining a healthy pregnancy and a trouble-free delivery, and they believe that working with their bodies in this way actually helps things go more smoothly. While there's not much medical evidence on the subject, I personally think that anything that makes a patient feel better helps. A hypnotist or psychotherapist may be able to help you learn more about visualization, or there are several books on the subject.

- **Meditation.** Meditation is a combination of deep breathing and a technique for clearing your mind of all thought. People who practice meditation find it deeply relaxing and energizing and claim that it helps them approach life in a more serene and joyous spirit. There's been some evidence that meditation is helpful in the treatment of migraine headache, which suggests that it has some power to help patients relax and possibly take a more positive attitude toward life. If meditation interests you, look for a book about it, or take a class at a local yoga center.

- **Massage.** Massage is relaxing, builds body awareness, and helps with the little aches, pains, and other discomforts that go with a multiple pregnancy. You can get a professional massage, teach your partner to massage you, or practice various kinds of self-massage. There are also several good books on massage that you and your partner might explore. By the way, many massage centers now offer special pregnancy massages, as well as featuring massage tables specially designed for pregnant women, with a hole in the table to put your belly in. Just be careful not to lie flat on your back for long periods of time, especially in the third trimester, and drink lots of fluids before and after your massage.

- **Journal writing.** Sometimes the best thing you can do for yourself is simply to listen—and one way to listen is to write down your thoughts and feelings without censoring anything. The important thing is to be honest and to know that your journal is private. Writing that you hate your partner, you wish you could kill your toddler, or that you sometimes would rather not be pregnant doesn't mean that you "really" feel that way, in the sense that you would ever take action to make any of these wishes come true. But acknowledging these wishes as one part of a complex bundle of emotions can be very liberating. You can also use your journal simply to muse about the changes that are happening in your life—or just to record your thoughts, with no particular agenda whatsoever.

Multiple Pregnancy and Your Sense of Self:
"I Don't Know Who I Am Anymore..."

You've probably noticed a common theme running through the previous discussion: When you're undergoing a multiple pregnancy, your sense of self is changing.

Of course, this makes sense. Before, you weren't a parent; now you will be. Or before, you were a parent of X number of children, but now you'll be a parent of X plus 2. You *are* becoming a different person, and while you're pregnant, you're also operating under different rules.

Many of us who get pregnant later in life—which includes lots of multiple moms—are used to having things our way. We've spent years getting good at our jobs, working out our relationships, building our social networks, and now we've got our lives pretty much the way we want them. Then we get pregnant with twins, or triplets, or quads, and all of a sudden we really are different people. The go-getter at work who prided herself on never being late with a presentation now has morning sickness and possibly bed rest to keep her from meeting her deadline. The superachiever who juggled friends, family, relationship, and job now feels as though she's dropped another ball every time she turns around.

For those of us who find it hard to relax, to let down, to feel needy or inadequate—and I certainly count myself in this number!—being pregnant with multiples can be a real education. Suddenly, we *can't* push our bodies in the same way—it's not good for us *or* the babies we're carrying. Suddenly, meeting all our commitments isn't just up to us—two (or three, or four) other people are involved too.

Does this mean you have to give up all your ambition, all of your friends, all of your old self, and settle down to be a twenty-first-century version of June Cleaver? No, of course not. I haven't done that, and none of the ambitious women I've treated has done that either. What we have had to do—and what you may have to do—is develop a sense of self that's more flexible than the one we once had. We've had to learn how to roll with the punches *while* setting high goals for ourselves, to let go and relax *while* striving and pushing hard.

You won't know ahead of time what this "new" self will look like—and you'll find that throughout pregnancy and parenthood, your sense of self keeps changing. But if you stay open to what you learn, pregnancy and parenthood can become, among other things, a journey of self-discovery. I urge you to learn all you can about how to enjoy the ride!

5.

Working with Your Doctor: What You Can and Should Expect

Marsha had always been one of my favorite patients. Bright, intense, articulate, and well-organized, she'd breeze into my office with fascinating stories about the international company she owned and managed. She'd describe her frequent business trips to oversee factories in Indonesia, her long meetings with local fashion designers, her complicated negotiations with rivals and colleagues around the world.

Then she got pregnant with twins. I'd seen many of my patients who were thrown, even overwhelmed, by the news of their multiple pregnancies—but not Marsha. Well-organized and thorough as usual, she showed up with an eight-page, single-spaced birth plan, detailing her proposed diet and exercise regime for the next nine months, what method she wanted me to use for delivery, and how long she expected to spend recovering before going back to work.

"But Marsha," I said tentatively. "We're going to have to wait and see how things develop. We *might* be able to follow this plan—it's terrific that you've thought so much about what you want—but things don't always turn out the way we expect, especially in a multiple pregnancy. You might have to take some time off, you might even have to spend some time in bed. I see you've got two vaginal deliveries planned, and I'd love to oblige—but we might have to consider a C-section—it's way too soon to tell."

Marsha stared at me, more bewildered than I'd ever seen her. For the first time in her life, she'd run into a situation that she *couldn't* plan ahead of time—at least, not to the extent that she was used to. Instead, she was going to have to trust in our doctor–patient relationship—a relationship that would find the two of us working things out together, every step of the way.

Who Should Deliver My Baby?

Here are some of the people you'll be considering as you choose your practitioner:

- **Ob/gyn.** An obstetrician/gynecologist is a doctor—like myself—who specializes in the care of women. Ob/gyns specialize in seeing women through pregnancy and childbirth as well as caring for women's health regarding menstruation, menopause, and their entire reproductive system.
- **Perinatologist.** This physician is somewhat more specialized than an ob/gyn, focusing primarily on high-risk pregnancies. A perinatologist might care directly for a woman during a complicated pregnancy or might just be available if the ob/gyn needs backup. He or she will be consulted by the ob/gyn if there are any complications, will perform the sonograms, and will conduct specialized tests or procedures.
- **Neonatologist.** This specialized doctor cares only for newborns—usually newborns in distress. Your hospital or birthing center will ideally have at least one neonatologist available for backup during your delivery, especially if you deliver prematurely. A specialist on this level won't be involved during the pregnancy itself but might be consulted in specific situations.
- **Midwife.** For centuries, pregnant women relied on midwives— nonmedical personnel who knew a great deal about babies, women's bodies, and the process of pregnancy. Today, in most states, midwives are licensed, and they usually have both nursing

degrees and a basic grounding in medical knowledge. However, most midwives won't accept patients with twins, and none will accept women pregnant with triplets or higher-order multiples. Midwives who do accept twin pregnancies will insist on having a doctor in the room or on the hospital floor during delivery.

Choosing a Practitioner

Your first task is to choose a practitioner—someone with whom you feel comfortable working out all of the unpredictable details of your multiple pregnancy, someone who has the level of expertise you need. To make this all-important choice, you'll want to consider some specific qualifications, which I'll discuss below. In the last analysis, though, your own instinct—and perhaps also your partner's—is your most valuable resource. One doctor might give you all the right answers and still not "feel" right; another physician may disagree with you and yet seem like a person you can trust. You'll have to decide for yourself what's important to you—and what's possible, given where you live, your financial circumstances, and your insurance situation.

Because any multiple pregnancy is by definition high-risk, you'll want to be sure that certain kinds of backup are available, precautions that might not be necessary if you were carrying a singleton. For example, if you're pregnant with twins or triplets, you may well decide to go with an ob/gyn (my own specialty, as it happens!). However, any ob/gyn caring for a multiple pregnancy should have access to a perinatologist, a doctor who specializes in high-risk pregnancies. If you're pregnant with quads or higher-order multiples, you should be seeing a perinatologist, at least for consultation.

Sonography

I would strongly recommend that your practitioner have easy access to sonography (a noninvasive method of viewing the fetuses via sonar). In my opinion, regular sonograms are indispensable in a multiple pregnancy: for monitoring the babies' growth, for discovering any anomalies or defects that might cause problems during the delivery, and for assuring that both babies are positioned in such a way that a vaginal delivery is possible. There's been some controversy over how necessary it is to administer routine sonograms for singleton pregnancies—but every responsible doctor agrees that multiple moms need regular sonograms. (For more on sonography, see Chapter 6.)

Hospital Facilities

Another key factor in choosing a practitioner is the kind of medical facilities to which he or she has access. Of course, your ob/gyn will be affiliated with a hospital—but what type of hospital? Since twins, triplets, and quads are more likely to be born prematurely, you want a doctor whose hospital includes a Level 3 nursery—a nursery qualified to handle early babies, including being able to resuscitate them. Otherwise, if there's an emergency, you might have to check into a hospital where your doctor can't practice, and you'll go through delivery with a doctor you've never met. Alternatively, you might find yourself giving birth in your doctor's hospital—and then risking an ambulance transfer of your tiny newborns to another place that's better equipped.

Many hospitals have separate birthing centers within the actual hospital facility, and this is a lovely option for a singleton. But it's far better to deliver twins in a place where your doctor has easy access to operating rooms. And I would strongly recommend against home delivery: Multiple pregnancies are just too risky, even when they go full-term. Multiple births bring a higher likelihood of cord prolapses (in which the umbilical cord slips down into the cervix or vaginal canal), fetal distress, and postpartum hemorrhage. If any of these conditions should arise, you want a hospital's resources close at hand.

What About Midwives?

In the last two decades, midwives have become increasingly popular with pregnant women. They can often spend more time with a pregnant woman than a doctor can, and they are committed to being with a woman throughout every minute of the birthing process—a commitment most doctors can't make. On the other hand, they have far less specialized knowledge than doctors, and there are many emergency procedures, most notably a cesarean section, that they simply cannot perform.

In my opinion, it's problematic to have a midwife deliver multiples because of the increased chances of a C-section or of fetal distress. Sometimes, even when Twin A is born smoothly, Twin B runs into unexpected problems—and since there's no way to know about this ahead of time, it's important to have medical personnel monitoring the situation.

These days, more and more women are turning to yet another type of help: a doula, someone (almost always a woman) whose job it is to provide various kinds of support during and after pregnancy. Doulas often accompany moms during a birth, supplementing the care of midwives, doctors, or even specialists, but not every health professional is comfortable having a doula present during delivery. If you want a doula in your hospital room, make sure you discuss the possibility with the doctor or midwife who will be supervising your birth.

To Specialize or Not to Specialize?

If you live in a large urban area, you might be considering a perinatologist as your primary-care provider during the pregnancy. While at first glance this may seem like the highest-quality option, be wary. Find out whether the specialist you have in mind is more interested in researching unusual cases than in the actual delivery of your twins. Ask how many multiples he or she personally delivers each year, and compare that number to what an experienced ob/gyn can offer. Find out whether your specialist will join you on the labor floor at night (which is when many deliveries take place), or if the doctor will be home in bed, leaving your care to a resident.

Of course, in complicated pregnancies or if you're carrying triplets or quads, a perinatologist should be available for consultation. But you may not wish to choose this type of specialist to supervise your pregnancy.

Doctor or Twin Clinic?

You might also be considering a so-called twin clinic, another type of specialized facility that focuses on multiple pregnancies. A twin clinic can offer you specialized, experienced care, but there might be some disadvantages. If you've established a good relationship with your ob/gyn, you'll be sacrificing the continuity of care you might otherwise have had, the chance to work with someone who knows you and your body very well. Also, if there's no twin clinic in your immediate vicinity, you might face the disruption and expense of travel. Some people have trouble getting their insurance to cover this level of care for what many insurance plans still see as a routine pregnancy. In any case, there are very few twin clinics.

Twin clinics do offer some distinct advantages: They have lots of experience with twins, and they follow certain principles of care that I believe are helpful. However, I personally believe that an experienced ob/gyn can offer the same benefits—*if* he or she sticks to those principles:

- consistent evaluation of the mother's symptoms and of her cervix;
- intensive education of patients about preterm labor (see Chapter 14);
- advice to the mother on modifying her activities as needed, such as reducing business travel, getting more rest, or, occasionally, undergoing bed rest;
- attention to the mother's nutrition and weight gain;
- follow-up on failed appointments;
- a warm, supportive environment that recognizes the multiple mom's unique needs.

Planning for an Emergency

What if you live in a geographic area where you don't have easy access to a Level 3 nursery, let alone a twin clinic? First of all, remember that there's a strong chance that you won't actually need this type of nursery. Your twin delivery might proceed easily with no complications, in which case your local hospital facilities may be just fine.

However, you should find out what kinds of emergency transportation are available. If you're in early labor, will they stabilize you and then transfer you, or will they deliver you and then transfer your babies? What does your doctor think of these arrangements? How comfortable do you feel with them? Is it practical to spend the last few months of your pregnancy in a place where you have access to better facilities? Bear in mind that as the mother of multiples, you're far more likely to deliver early. Bear in mind, too, that you don't want to be driving long distances toward the end of your pregnancy—and certainly not during labor! Because you're carrying multiples, you'll want to plan for emergencies to a greater extent than if you were pregnant with a singleton.

Weighing Your Options

As you can see, there's no one best option when it comes to choosing a doctor. It's a juggling act, in which you'll weigh several options and decide what's most important to you. To summarize, here are the questions you'll want to ask:

- How experienced with multiples is the person who will be delivering me?
- How comfortable do I feel with my practitioner and with the environment in which I'll be delivering?
- Does my practitioner have access to consultation and sonography?
- Do I have access to an adequate nursery in case of premature delivery?
- If I have to be transported to a regional hospital or birthing center, what kind of transportation is available?

The Obstetrical Balancing Act

As an ob/gyn who has herself gone through three pregnancies, I've seen the doctor–patient relationship from both sides of the examination table. As a patient, I want to be able to call my doctor at the drop of a hat, to hear her reassurance whenever I need it. As a doctor, I understand that if all my patients came into the office every time they had a question, my practice would grind to a halt. As a patient, I, too, worry about what might go wrong. As a doctor, I try to practice what I think of as the *art* of obstetrics: striking the balance between being overly reassuring and making the patient feel she has to rush in to my office at the least little sign of something unusual.

As the patient in a relatively high-risk pregnancy, it may be helpful for you to think of the patient–doctor relationship as a balancing act in which both you and your physician are finding your way. You do need to be more alert to signs of preterm labor, but such alertness need not necessarily mean more anxiety. Like Marsha, you'll have to negotiate a path between taking no thought at all for the future and having an overly certain idea of how you want your delivery to proceed. As I keep discovering, making plans and then having them *not* work out is probably the best preparation for parenthood there is!

A Doctor–Patient Bill of Rights

So what *is* reasonable to expect from your practitioner—and what should he or she expect from you? In the final analysis, only *you* can make this decision. But here are a couple of sample checklists to help you think through the process:

Your doctor should . . .
- feel accessible to you;
- respect your time;
- be receptive to your ideas about the kind of health care you want, including the ways you want your partner involved in the delivery;
- be able to communicate to you and your partner with respect, even when you disagree;
- set clear guidelines for how often he or she wants to see you during your pregnancy;
- have an acceptable (that is, acceptable to you!) way of handling and returning your phone calls and of distinguishing between

which questions can be handled by phone, which can wait for your regular visit, and which require an emergency visit;

- have acceptable backup people whom you see if he or she is not available;
- be experienced in handling multiple births;
- have admitting privileges at a hospital with a Level 3 nursery and have a perinatologist available for consultation.

You should . . .
- respect your doctor's time;
- take responsibility for noticing what's happening to your body and use good judgment in reporting that to your doctor;
- fully disclose your employment situation; travel plans; exercise patterns; eating habits; use of vitamins, minerals, and herbal supplements; drug and alcohol use, including over-the-counter drugs and prescribed medications; sexual activity; and any other information that your doctor feels is necessary to monitor your pregnancy;
- be proactive in learning about your pregnancy and in making decisions about treatment;
- be flexible and mindful of the fact that neither you nor your doctor can completely control how your pregnancy and delivery proceeds;
- follow agreed-upon treatments that your doctor prescribes or suggests, and report openly and fully any times you *don't* follow such treatments.

The day I told Marsha that her birth plan might not work was a real test of our relationship. She needed to trust that I had her interests and her babies' interests at heart; I needed to respect her wish to make her own decisions about this momentous event in her life. As we proceeded through her pregnancy, our relationship would continue to be tested. Every time an unexpected development occurred, the two of us wrestled with how to respond. Could I help her fit this new occurrence into her life, or should I be telling her that her life had to change? Could she remain committed to her career without endangering her pregnancy, or did she have to accept a level of compromise that she had never expected to face?

Marsha *did* trust me, and I respected her. Despite a number of complications, we worked together toward her successful delivery of two healthy baby boys at a respectable six pounds each at 35 weeks. For Marsha, as it will be for you, the key was communication and knowledge. Know what you want, be willing to talk about it, and be open to listening to what your doctor has to say. With goodwill and mutual respect, you, your partner, and your doctor can forge a strong partnership to ease the journey through pregnancy and delivery.

6.

Making Choices: Prenatal Diagnosis, Prenatal Decisions

In some ways, your multiple pregnancy is like a long road with a number of important signposts and tricky turning points. In this chapter, we'll look at some of the choices that you'll face along the road.

Sonograms

We talked about the first big signpost in Chapter 4—diagnosing that you're pregnant with more than one fetus. Your doctor probably made or confirmed this diagnosis with a *sonogram,* or *ultrasound,* which uses sonar waves to create an image of your unborn children.

Besides establishing that you have a multiple pregnancy, a sonogram helps to establish your due date. This is especially important in a multiple pregnancy, since preterm labor and premature birth are so common for twins, triplets, and quads. If you go into preterm labor, the doctor needs to know exactly how long you've been pregnant, to decide how aggressively to intervene.

Sonograms have become a routine part of most U.S. pregnancies these days, and they are even more common in multiple pregnancies. However, this is a controversial area. Although everyone agrees that sonograms are perfectly safe, there's been a lot of debate over whether it's necessary to use them routinely. On the *con* side are the arguments that regular sonograms "overmedicalize" a pregnancy and that they add an expense and inconvenience that may not improve outcomes. On the *pro* side are the arguments that sonograms help doctors identify problems much earlier than they otherwise could, as well as helping to establish an accurate due date.

Let's look at the discussion a little more closely. The most famous "anti-sonogram" argument came out of the famous RADIUS trial, a study of Routine Antenatal (prebirth) Diagnostic Imaging with Ultrasound—that is, a study of the routine use of ultrasound. In its far-reaching study of U.S. pregnancies, the RADIUS survey included 129 multiple pregnancies. The study found that routine use of ultrasound did indeed lead to an earlier diagnosis of multiple pregnancies. (Today, thanks to ultrasound, fewer than 10 percent of all twins go undiagnosed, whereas in 1970, the figure was closer to 50 percent.)

However, the RADIUS study also found that better diagnosis was not necessarily associated with better outcomes. The rates of premature birth, complications, miscarriage, and stillbirth were just as high among women who were given frequent sonograms as among those who didn't have routine ultrasound. And, of course, the routine ultrasound made the pregnancies far more expensive.

Since then, other studies have contradicted RADIUS, showing that there are indeed fewer neonatal (newborn) deaths when sonograms are used early in the pregnancy.

How can we evaluate this controversy? Well, first, we have to consider a major criticism of the RADIUS study: that the sonograms it studied were simply not done very well. Many observers, myself included, believe that if the sonograms had been done by more-competent personnel, they would have picked up more fetal abnormalities, allowing physicians to alter their treatment plans as needed. Had this been done, the study would have shown that routine sonography does indeed lead to improved outcomes—that is, to fewer complications and a better survival rate for mothers and infants.

And let's remember the one thing that everyone agrees upon: Routine ultrasound means that you're far more likely to find out whether you're carrying a multiple pregnancy.

Other than to make an initial diagnosis, why is routine ultrasound important? In my opinion, for several reasons:

- **To create a prenatal-care plan based on the risks known to occur at various ages of the fetus.** If I can follow a multiple pregnancy closely with regular sonograms, I can watch out for congenital anomalies, poor or uneven growth of the fetuses, and the possibility of preterm labor.
- **To determine the type of twinning, including the number of placentas, amnions, and chorions.** As you recall from Chapter 3, the type of twinning makes a huge difference in how the pregnancy and delivery progress. Knowing whether the twins are monochorionic or dichorionic helps me assess how risky the birth is likely to be and to prepare for the appropriate treatments if complications should arise. For example, up to 50 percent of women carrying monoamniotic twins lose one or both of their babies before delivery. If your twins are sharing an amnion, your doctor will want to keep a very close eye on your condition. Likewise, a monochorionic-diamniotic pregnancy has a higher risk of twin–twin transfusion syndrome, a condition in which one twin grows at the expense of the other. If this is your type of pregnancy, your doctor will monitor the growth of each twin with special care, and you may be referred to a perinatal unit with special expertise in managing these conditions, either for consultation or for a specialist to take over your case.
- **To evaluate the amount of fetal amniotic fluid.** Either too much or too little can mean problems.
- **To detect any abnormalities in the placenta.** Again, such abnormalities might pose problems in the pregnancy or birth, so I like to know about them as early as possible. For example, one of my patients pregnant with twins developed early third-trimester bleeding, which the sonogram revealed to be coming from a

blood vessel on the placental plate. A timely C-section enabled us to deliver two feisty, 4½-pound baby girls.

- **To monitor the growth of each fetus.** If your twins are suffering from twin–twin transfusion syndrome, the best way to find out is through routine ultrasound. In addition, up to one-third of all twins suffer from some kind of fetal growth restriction. Routine ultrasound gives me a chance to find out about such problems as early as possible and, hopefully, to take steps to address them. For example, if the babies aren't growing properly, the mother may need to restrict her activity or even to consider bed rest. In severe cases of twin–twin transfusion syndrome, we might want to consider delivering the babies earlier than we otherwise would, through induced labor or a C-section, or to respond with some other active intervention (for more about twin–twin transfusion, see Chapter 13).

- **To watch for fetal anomalies, particularly those unique to twins.** There's a higher rate of chromosomal and structural problems with twins, up to 1 in 50, especially monozygotic ("identical") twins. Some 7 percent of all dizygotic twins suffer from anomalies, versus 3 percent of singletons. And several conditions unique to twins can be detected only by a sonogram: for example, an acardiac twin (where one of the twins has no heart), conjoined twins (popularly if inaccurately known as "Siamese twins"), vanishing-twin syndrome (the loss of one twin), and twin–twin transfusion syndrome. Diagnosing these problems in the second trimester helps both me and the parents manage the pregnancy, assess the risks of delivery, and prepare to care properly for the newborns.

Most important, in my opinion, is the need to prevent preterm labor and premature birth, which is far more common among multiple pregnancies than among singletons. (For more on this topic, see Chapter 14.) So if I know that a woman is pregnant with twins—knowledge that I can most reliably get from routine ultrasound—I'll be on the lookout for signs of preterm labor and I'll prepare the mother for ways she can help prevent it. She may need to modify her lifestyle, eat differently, or make other adjustments—but we won't know that unless we know she's expecting twins. We may also be able to diagnose the chances of delivering prematurely by measuring the mother's cervical length via sonogram, in addition to palpating the cervix (see Chapter 15).

I hope I've convinced you that you should be getting regular sonograms to monitor your pregnancy! Of course, this is something that you and your doctor will have to decide together. But you should be certain that you and your physician share the same philosophy on this important issue.

Facing a Loss

Just as women who are pregnant with singletons face the possibility of miscarriage or loss of the fetus, so do women who are pregnant with multiples run the risk of losing one or more of their babies. In fact, up to 50 percent of twin gestations diagnosed early in the first trimester do not result in the delivery of two live infants.

When a twin pregnancy, diagnosed by sonogram, is lost early in the first trimester, that is known as the vanishing-twin syndrome. This loss may be evident only on the ultrasound, as vaginal spotting or bleeding occurs in only about 25 percent of these cases.

Although figures vary, one study found that over 20 percent of all twin pregnancies were marked by early loss of one twin—about the same spontaneous loss rate as for singleton pregnancies. Another study found that 25 percent of all multiple pregnancies resulting from ART included the loss of a twin, triplet, or quad.

It's generally agreed that the mother suffers no physical problems from a first-trimester loss and that the prognosis for the surviving twin, triplets, or quads is excellent. After the first trimester, loss of a fetus becomes more serious—and less likely. Only 2 to 5 percent of all twin pregnancies lose one fetus after the third month, although the figure is somewhat higher for triplets—14 to 17 percent.

Losses are three to four times higher for monochorionic twins than for dichorionic babies. That's because twins sharing a chorion are less insulated from each other. For all types of twins, of course, a loss later in gestation means that the surviving twin must be monitored closely throughout the pregnancy.

What's the Prognosis?

Although it's often impossible to predict the loss of a twin, there are some indicators that your doctor will be looking out for. A congenital or structural anomaly in one or more fetuses might indicate that the fetus will have trouble surviving. This is a particular concern for parents of multiples, because, as we saw earlier, congenital anomalies are more common among twins.

However, even when twins are monozygotic, only one twin may be affected by an anomaly. Or both may be affected, but only one severely. Dizygotic twins, of course, have separate genetic inheritances and are no more likely to share an anomaly than two siblings born at different times.

Hard Choices: Reducing a Pregnancy with Anomalies

Cheryl was 38 years old. She'd been trying to get pregnant for over two years, and finally, by taking Pergonal and using IVF, she'd conceived twin boys. She and her husband, Don, were delighted—and dismayed. Cheryl and her husband were both Fragile X carriers, and she had a mildly retarded brother whose condition had apparently been caused by the Fragile X syndrome. "I love my brother, but I saw how hard it was for my mother," she told me. "And Don has never felt comfortable with him—I'm not happy about that, but it's true. I'm honestly not sure that we're the right parents for even one special-needs child, let alone two."

Cheryl decided that before making any decisions, she had to find out more. At ten weeks, she had CVS (chorionic villus sampling), which revealed that one of her fetuses was indeed affected by Fragile X, though the other was not. The fetus affected by Fragile X might be born anywhere on the spectrum from mildly learning disabled to severely retarded.

Cheryl and Don were facing some hard choices. Did they want to accept the pregnancy and hope for the best? Would they consider "reducing" the pregnancy—terminating only the fetus with Fragile X? Would the surviving child feel like a constant reminder of the missing twin? Did they want to abort the entire pregnancy and try again? None of the choices felt easy—but as Cheryl's first trimester proceeded, they knew they had to make a choice.

I explained to Cheryl and Don that fetal reduction poses at least a five percent risk of losing the entire pregnancy. There's also a slightly higher risk of delivering prematurely after a reduction, so if they did decide to reduce part of their pregnancy, Cheryl would be undergoing ultrasound to monitor her closely for signs of preterm labor: a shortening cervix, or fetal membranes "funneling" into the birth canal. In the past, doctors used to think that reduction also led to increased risk of growth restriction for the remaining fetuses, but we now see that this seems to occur only when reducing from more than four fetuses.

Eventually Cheryl and Don decided to proceed with the pregnancy and hope for the best, and Cheryl delivered two healthy boys at 35 weeks. The baby affected by Fragile X seemed alert, though his parents won't know for many years whether he has learning disabilities or to what extent they'll affect him.

Hard Choices: Reducing a Normal Multiple Pregnancy

If a triplet or quad pregnancy includes only healthy fetuses, parents may face another hard choice: whether to reduce the number of fetuses in order to protect the health of the mother and/or the remaining fetuses. This is a complicated decision that involves weighing the mother's health, the number of fetuses involved, the condition of the fetuses, and the parents' philosophical and religious outlook. Ideally, women considering this choice would get counseling both from doctors who have performed reductions and from doctors and neonatologists who have delivered and cared for multiple fetuses.

With quads and higher-order multiples, it's clear that reducing to triplets or twins vastly increases the babies' chance of survival. Reducing otherwise healthy triplets to twins is not so clear-cut. Twins tend to be born later than triplets and at higher birth weights, which increases their chances for survival and improves their health. Even twins who do suffer problems are likely to have shorter stays than triplets in the neonatal intensive-care unit (NICU). There is also a drop in the triplet pregnancy's loss rate with a reduction from three to two (approximately 15 percent to approximately 5 percent). The reduced twins fared similarly to nonreduced twins. Mothers had fewer major illnesses associated with pregnancy, such as preeclampsia and postpartum hemorrhaging, and tended to spend fewer days in the hospital, which also reduced the cost of their pregnancy. And there was a decrease in the "moderate morbidities" (moderate illnesses) associated with prolonged hospital stays and preterm deliveries.

However, with improvements in prenatal care, an ongoing triplet pregnancy can result in excellent outcomes. In other words, even if triplets and their mothers had to stay in the hospital longer, possibly running up a higher bill and getting moderately sick in the process, they were eventually just as likely to go home healthy as were families with twins. Clearly, this is a highly personal decision.

Reducing otherwise-healthy triplets to a singleton or two healthy fetuses to one is a controversial procedure, and there's no evidence that it increases the chances of mother or infant survival any more than reducing triplets to twins. Therefore, some doctors and hospitals choose not to perform it and feel it is not ethical. Others feel that such a decision should be the parents' choice, just as with abortion, and tell patients that they will be less likely to have a cesarean section, and may carry the pregnancy two or three weeks longer.

Finding Out More

Clearly, it's to your advantage to find out as soon as possible whether one or more of your multiples has a fetal anomaly. If termination and reduction are options for you, you'll want to make that decision as soon as possible. If these procedures are not options, you and your doctor will still want to be prepared for the complications that fetal anomalies can bring, as well as be prepared for the delivery and care of the affected fetuses.

Of course, every test brings with it risks as well as benefits. For

example, many tests used to diagnose fetal defects themselves pose
some risk to the pregnancy. A couple who for personal or religious
reasons would not abort an "abnormal" child might be especially un-
willing to risk certain tests.

For singletons, chromosomal testing is recommended if the
mother is over 35 or the father is over 50. In a multiple pregnancy, because of the higher rate of chromosomal abnormalities, the recommended age is lower for the mother: 32 or 33 for twins, and 31 in the
case of triplets. You might also want to consider chromosomal testing
by CVS or amniocentesis if:

- you have an abnormal ultrasound;
- your screening turns up an abnormality;
- your family history or previous pregnancies indicate a pattern of
  certain problems;
- your genetic history indicates that you and/or your partner is a
  carrier of some genetic condition.

What Tests Are Available?

Let's say you have good reason to be concerned that one or more of
your multiples has some kind of abnormality and you want to find
out more. What kinds of tests can you have?

The first test to consider is CVS, or a chorionic villus sampling.
Like amniocentesis, it's used to check for chromosomal abnormalities
and genetic diseases, such as Down's syndrome, Tay-Sachs, sickle-cell
anemia, most types of cystic fibrosis, and thalassemia (see Chapter 2).

As Cheryl and Don found out, CVS can be done as early as the
10th to 12th week, whereas amniocentesis isn't usually done until 15
to 18 weeks. CVS—performed at certain medical centers only—
involves a needle inserted into the abdominal wall (*transabdominal CVS*)
or a catheter inserted into the vagina and cervix (*transcervical CVS*) in
order to take a sample of the placental tissue. Both versions of the procedure may cause mild discomfort and cramping for a short time.

Although amniocentesis is a relatively simple procedure, it can be
rather dramatic to witness. I'll never forget the time I performed an
amniocentesis on Tanya, a 35-year-old nurse who was calm and col-

The Limits of Testing

When I test women for fetal problems, I try to make clear the limits of the testing procedure. But sometimes all of us wish so hard for clear, certain answers that these explanations fall short. Trying to be reassuring, a doctor may make some results sound more encouraging and definite than they are. Fearing the worst, a mother-to-be may worry needlessly over a result that indicates only a probability, not a certainty.

Think of a test literally as a screening procedure—as a wire mesh stretched over a wooden frame. Information about you and your babies is "poured" through the mesh. If the mesh catches something and won't let it pass through, that's a "positive" result, suggesting that, say, a baby has increased risk of Down's syndrome or spina bifida. If the mesh catches nothing, that's a "negative" result, suggesting that the baby is free from the defect or problem that was being screened for.

As I hope this metaphor makes clear, screening is far from a foolproof process. Some positive problems fall through the mesh and don't show up until the baby is actually born. Some misinformation can get caught by the mesh, suggesting that there is a problem when actually everything is fine.

It's often not possible to design the ideal screen—one that "catches" all the positives without including the negatives. Even when it's medically possible to create such a test, it's often prohibitively expensive; a test that includes some false positives while catching all (or almost all) the actual positives may be far more affordable. Such a test may also be less invasive and easier to administer.

There are some exciting new tests on the horizon, such as the *fetal nuchal translucency test* with accompanying early serum (blood) screening, which will possibly detect birth defects far earlier in the course of pregnancy and with less risk to the fetus. Unfortunately, these tests' effectiveness outside the United Kingdom—where they've been developed—has yet to be established conclusively. However, a large U.S. study is currently under way. Meanwhile, we'll continue with the tests we now have—giving thanks for the blessings of modern medical technology while cautioning our patients to beware of the limits of testing.

lected in what was, to her, a familiar medical setting. However, her tall and strapping husband saw me inserting the needle into Tanya's abdominal wall—and passed out. Luckily, there was a nurse on hand to take care of *him*! Ever since this experience, I make a point of keeping an eye on the partner's color—and I always have a chair available!

CVS is somewhat harder to perform on multiples than on singletons. It's more difficult to obtain an adequate sample, and it's harder to keep one sample from contaminating the other. About one percent of all women who have CVS lose one or both babies—so if you are committed to carrying your entire pregnancy to term, no matter how many fetuses you have or what their condition, you probably won't want this test.

On the other hand, if you are considering reduction—say, if you discover that one twin is abnormal and the other is not—you will want the chance to have the procedure done as soon as possible, so that there will be less risk of complication. Also, in rare cases, CVS enables fetal therapy to be performed at an earlier date.

Amniocentesis also has a loss rate of about 1 percent, but you must wait until the 15th to 18th week before you have it. For women considering termination or reduction, this longer wait may not be acceptable.

Amniocentesis also involves using a needle to extract samples—in this case, samples of amniotic fluid from each fetus's sac. Usually, after fluid from the first sac is taken, some carmine-indigo dye is injected back in, so that the second fetus's fluid is clear by contrast. However, in the case of monozygotic twins, only one sac needs to be tapped, as it's extremely rare for the fetuses to have different genetic material.

Knowing the Situation

If you are considering a pregnancy reduction, you will want to know which, if any, fetuses have chromosomal abnormalities or other birth defects. You may want to have CVS before any reduction is performed, so that the person performing the CVS can make a careful map of each fetus's location, allowing the abnormal fetus(es) to be targeted for reduction. Ideally, the same person would both conduct the

CVS and reduce the fetuses, since he or she would be most familiar with the "geography" of the pregnancy.

After CVS, you may still want a blood sample taken in the 15th to 18th week of your pregnancy for *maternal serum screening*. This test measures the alpha-fetoprotein (the fetal protein) in the mother's blood as well as other markers such as human chorionic gonadotropin (hCG) and unconjugated estriol (sometimes called a triple screen). Maternal serum alpha-fetoprotein (MSAFP) is produced by fetuses, and high levels of it in your blood are one sign that you're carrying more than one fetus. If you had a reduction, your MSAFP levels will certainly be elevated, so they won't be measured.

Sometimes, high levels of MSAFP indicate a neural-tube defect, such as spina bifida (a defect in the spinal column), anencephaly (in which all or part of the brain is absent—a condition that is almost always picked up on the ultrasound), or other abnormalities. In single-ton pregnancies, abnormally low levels of MSAFP, along with other markers, can indicate Down's syndrome or another chromosomal abnormality, but this is not a reliable indicator with multiples.

Clearly, if you're carrying a multiple pregnancy, your MSAFP will be elevated. In fact, one of the ways that twins can be diagnosed is by this elevation. Therefore, this test is less useful for detecting abnormalities in twins and not useful at all for triplets or higher-order multiples. However, if your first MSAFP screening is more than 4.5 times the median, you may be carrying a structurally abnormal fetus. Although the data is inconclusive, a detailed sonogram and perhaps also an amniocentesis will then be performed.

Mourning and Moving On

What if you do decide to reduce your pregnancy, terminating one or two of the fetuses you are carrying? Even if you know this is the best decision for you and your family, you may still be deeply affected by the loss. Likewise, if you've been pregnant with quads, triplets, or twins and one or more fetuses spontaneously miscarry, you may feel a sense of loss even though you're still pregnant.

One of my patients had tried unsuccessfully for a long time to conceive. Finally, she and her husband tried IVF, and she became pregnant with a singleton, which she successfully delivered. A second use of IVF led to a twin pregnancy, which made her very happy. At about ten weeks, one of the twins spontaneously miscarried. The other, though, was fine, and my patient seemed relieved and happy—almost too happy. She claimed that she was just as glad not to have to deal with twins and that her main feeling was joy at this miraculous second pregnancy.

All seemed to be well—until the weeks after she finally delivered. Although her new baby was healthy and beautiful, my patient suffered a crushing postpartum depression. It seemed to me that she had needed to mourn the vanishing twin—even if she really did prefer to have only one new baby. By moving too quickly away from the mourning period, she had opened herself to renewed grief later on.

Another one of my patients was pregnant with triplets, which she seemed willing to carry. Her husband, however, was absolutely certain that he couldn't handle three children at once—neither financially nor emotionally—and he convinced her to reduce the pregnancy to a single child. My patient insisted that she had made the right decision for herself, her child, and her marriage. Yet every time she came in for a checkup, she burst into tears. Clearly, she had some feelings about the reduction that she had not yet dealt with. It may indeed have been the right decision for her, or she might have acted under pressure. Either way, she needed to acknowledge and mourn her loss.

As you consider your own marital, financial, and emotional situation, you, too, may be faced with hard choices about prenatal diagnosis. I urge you to make sure you fully understand all the medical issues involved and then to discuss your decision with anyone who might be supportive—your doctor, your partner, a relative or friend, even a professional counselor. Whatever you decide, give your decision the respect it deserves and allow yourself all the time you need to ponder, mourn, and celebrate your choice.

7.

Creating Healthy Babies:
Nutrition

✍

Too often, people believe that a multiple pregnancy is pretty much like any other. In fact, the special demands and high stakes involved in multiple pregnancy call for multiple moms to go that extra mile. Any pregnancy requires certain changes in your work life, home routine, eating habits, and exercise patterns—but because your risks are higher, your pregnancy will require more changes than most.

In this chapter, I'll focus on nutrition: how much weight to gain and the best way to gain it. I'll also talk about vitamins, minerals, and supplements—the ones to take and the ones to avoid. In Chapter 8, we'll talk about medications—what you can't take, what you should take—and in Chapter 9, exercise and bed rest.

Early, Adequate Weight Gain

Remember Shana and Rosario from Chapter 2? Shana, a runway model, embarked on her multiple pregnancy at about 20 pounds under her optimal weight, while Rosario, a social worker, was about 20 pounds heavier than we thought she should be.

EARLY, ADEQUATE WEIGHT GAIN:
THE BEST GIFT YOU CAN GIVE

Mother's optimal weight gain:	24th week	37th week
Pregnant with Singleton	12–15 pounds	25–35 pounds
Pregnant with Twins	24–30 pounds	50 pounds

Both women, however, shared a common task: to make sure they enjoyed *early, adequate weight gain,* so that their unborn multiples would be well-nourished and prepared for the possibility of premature birth.

Let's be clear about this: We're not just talking about the total weight gain over the course of the pregnancy. If you've been pregnant before, or if you've closely observed your pregnant friends and relatives, you've probably noticed that normal-weight women carrying singletons gain most of their weight in the second trimester. In most cases, they're gaining from half a pound to a pound per week, for an eventual total of about 30 pounds.

The mother of twins, on the other hand, needs to gain more—usually at least 40 pounds, acquired at the rate of at least a pound a week—and she needs to gain more of that weight in the first trimester. That's because twins in general are likely to be born earlier than singletons, and they're more likely to be born prematurely. The best resource a premature baby has is birth weight—so unborn twins need to be well and fully nourished pretty much from the moment of conception.

Of course, early, adequate weight gain is even more important for the mothers of triplets, quads, and higher-order multiples. These babies are even more likely to be born early, giving them even less time inside you to grow and develop. Their best chance of survival is a healthy birth weight—which you must begin to build up as early as possible in the pregnancy.

Underweight, Overweight, or Normal Weight?

Women like Shana who start their multiple pregnancies underweight may need to gain more weight more quickly. One study found that underweight women who gained more than a pound a week before Week 20 and more than 1.75 pounds a week *after* Week 20 were likely to have twins weighing 2,500 grams, or 5½ pounds each, an optimal outcome!

If normal-weight women wanted that same, positive outcome, the study found, they needed to gain at least 1½ pounds a week after Week 20.

Overweight women, like Rosario, may need to curtail their weight gain during pregnancy, in order to counter the increased risk of high blood pressure, pregnancy-induced diabetes, and the need to deliver by C-section. However, most women think of themselves as fatter than they really are—so once again, I urge you to talk to your doctor!

There's another reason why multiple moms gain extra weight. When you're carrying twins, you have not only two babies within you, but also two placentas and a still greater increase of blood and amniotic fluid. If you're pregnant with triplets, quads, or higher-order multiples, you have even more to carry—and your ideal weight goes up accordingly.

Of course, your optimal weight gain will vary depending on whether you began your pregnancy overweight, underweight, or at your "ideal" weight. So in the final analysis, what you "should" weigh at each stage of pregnancy is a number best determined by you and your doctor. However, you should know that multiple moms who have a *low* rate of early weight gain—less than 21 pounds, or less than 0.85 pounds per week before Week 24—are more likely to have babies whose prenatal growth is slowed and who are more at risk for other prenatal problems.

Shana was horrified when I told her about the weight gain she should be aiming for. "Dr. Leiter," she told me, almost in tears. "All my life I've fought to keep my weight down. It's not just an ego thing—it's part of my job! Now you're telling me I have to gain more than a pound a week? I'll feel awful carrying all that extra fat around—and I'll spend my whole pregnancy worrying about how I'm going to lose it!"

While most of my patients don't have the professional reasons to stay thin that Shana did, many of them are concerned about looking trim and slim. Like Shana, many of them felt that they'd spent their lives fighting each extra unwanted pound. While some women receive my nutritional counseling with joy—finally, an excuse to *gain* weight!—many others share Shana's dismay.

If you, too, look with horror upon the prospect of gaining pregnancy weight, I urge you to find ways of supporting a new body image, one that celebrates your ability to nurture your twins, triplets, or quads rather than one requiring you to fit society's standards of thinness. Talk about the issue with your partner, supportive friends, or a counselor; treat yourself to a luxurious massage that reminds you of how much pleasure your body can give you; surround yourself with prints of Rubens nudes or sensuous photographs of pregnant women. Your babies really *need* you to gain weight, so any way that you can find to enjoy the process will help you all.

Rosario, on the other hand, was dismayed for a different reason: I had explained to her that if she gained too much weight too quickly, she'd be at greater risk for high blood pressure, preeclampsia, gestational diabetes (diabetes set off by pregnancy), and other conditions. "All I have to do is look at a French fry, and I gain," she told me. "Diets don't seem to help—they never have. And now that I'm pregnant, I'm hungry all the time."

If you, too, are working with your doctor to control your weight gain, let me urge you to find the support *you* need. Maybe a nutritionist can help you come up with delicious but less-fattening snacks; perhaps a pregnancy support group can help; you might discover that a mild exercise regime—one that suits your multiple-pregnant condition—makes a crucial difference.

Either way, try to be gentle with yourself. Issues around weight are extremely charged for most women in our society, regardless of what they actually weigh. Staying in touch with your feelings and reaching out for support can help you make your way gracefully through this process. And you can always take off some of those pregnancy pounds by nursing your newborns!

Morning Sickness, Heartburn, and Other Delights

All right, so how do you acquire these extra pounds in the healthiest possible way? And how can you even *think* about eating with the extra-intense "morning sickness" that usually accompanies a multiple pregnancy?

Morning sickness, as you may already have found out, is poorly named, for it can happen at any time of the day. Estimates of how many women experience nausea and vomiting during pregnancy range from 40 to 50 percent in one study of Australian women to 88 percent in an American study.

What causes morning sickness? No one knows, though it seems to be associated with changing hormones in your body, including hCG, the pregnancy hormone, and thyroxine. Elevated progesterone levels may also contribute to some nausea and vomiting by decreasing your stomach's muscle tone and slowing its *motility* (ability to move food through the stomach). At the same time, your pregnant stomach gets bigger inside. These three factors make it hard for your stomach to empty completely, which tends to make you nauseous. Thus morning sickness is most likely to happen when your stomach is relatively empty—such as when you wake up in the morning—since that's when stomach acids collect around the "leftover" food.

Because multiple moms have a higher level of the pregnancy hormone in their blood, they tend to experience even more nausea and vomiting than singleton mothers do. Emotional factors can also cause nausea and vomiting to occur more frequently, with more severity, or both—so again, stressed-out multiple moms may experience more stomach upset.

Meanwhile, like many pregnant women, you may find that your central nervous system is more sensitive to odors—which you experience as a heightened sense of smell. That plus the morning sickness means that many foods you once enjoyed now tend to make you sick. You may find it difficult to prepare food for yourself, especially if you're cooking while you're hungry. Some women have even

When Morning Sickness Seems Out of Control...

It's rare for nausea and vomiting during pregnancy to pose a life-threatening problem—but it happens. About 1.3 percent of all pregnant women with nausea and vomiting need to be hospitalized to prevent the dehydration and malnutrition that can result. Neurological problems, liver and kidney damage, and retinal hemorrhage are also sometimes associated.

In these extreme cases, hospitalization allows you to be given antiemetics (drugs to control vomiting), administered through your rectum or via an intravenous (IV) or subcutaneous (SQ) pump. Home IV therapy is also gaining in popularity, as are home IV and SQ pumps for antinausea medications in severe cases.

Sometimes nausea and vomiting are symptoms of other health-threatening conditions, such as appendicitis, hepatitis, colitis, or food poisoning, which your doctor should diagnose and treat immediately. In rare cases, excessive nausea and vomiting indicate an abnormal pregnancy, such as an ectopic pregnancy (a pregnancy in which the egg is implanted elsewhere than in the uterus), which can be diagnosed by ultrasound.

reported feeling sick at "intense visual stimuli"—such as the lovingly photographed food in a TV commercial.

Morning sickness comes in two varieties:

- **"Normal" nausea and vomiting**—a mild-to-moderate condition. At this level, morning sickness doesn't result in dehydration, and even women who suffer from it experience some periods without it.
- **Hyperemesis gravidarium**—a far more rare—and severe—condition. (*Emesis* means *vomiting,* while *hyper* means *too much. Gravidarium* refers to pregnancy; thus, *pregnancy-related severe vomiting.*) The serious vomiting of hyperemesis can lead to dehydration, electrolyte imbalance, and weight loss. Some estimates find that

up to 6 percent of all pregnant women experience hyperemesis, while others place the figure far lower. There's also some evidence that this condition is less frequent now than it was 20 or 30 years ago.

To cheer you up, keep in mind that there are better outcomes with pregnancies that involve morning sickness, including fewer miscarriages and perinatal deaths. Animal and human studies show that there may even be a role for this misery in stimulating early placental growth.

Riding Out the Morning Sickness

"I actually didn't have problems with morning sickness the first two times I got pregnant," Zoe told me. "But those were singletons. I just wasn't prepared for how intense the vomiting and nausea would be when I was carrying triplets."

In most singleton pregnancies, vomiting tends to peak at about seven or eight weeks. In your case, you may be in for a longer, more intense period of nausea, but you're likely to be fine by the second trimester. Meanwhile, be sure to call your doctor if you are ever unable to hold food down for more than 24 hours. Likewise, if you aren't urinating much, feel dizzy or light-headed, or sense that your pulse is racing, call your doctor immediately, as you may be suffering from dehydration.

Heartburn and Indigestion

These twin problems will probably plague you throughout your pregnancy, more often and more severely than for mothers of singletons. Besides decreasing stomach tone, your increased progesterone levels are playing havoc with your *lower esophageal sphincter* (muscular ring)—the place where your esophagus joins your stomach—making that muscle less efficient. As your pregnancy proceeds, you've got more pressure on your abdomen. In response, your inefficient sphincter may allow some of the contents of your stomach—leftover food mixed with digestive acids—to push back up into your esophagus. The acid causes heartburn—heartburn that comes even earlier and more frequently during a twin pregnancy, since your extra-large uterus is putting even more pressure on your abdomen.

"I'd always loved exotic, spicy foods," Natalie recalls. "But it seemed like with every week of my pregnancy, I cut something else out of my diet. By the time the twins were born, I was practically living on brown rice, fish, hard-boiled eggs, and veggies—plus my four big glasses of milk each day!"

"Graze Like a Cow": Staying Nourished and Hydrated

As a multiple mom facing heartburn, indigestion, and nausea, you've got to be especially careful to stay well-hydrated. Of course, taking in enough protein, calcium, and other nutrients can be a challenge if you don't feel like eating.

I always tell my patients to "graze like a cow": to eat small amounts several times a day. Think in terms of small, frequent feedings or periodic snacks. Carry a water bottle with you—especially if it's summer, or if you've been vomiting—and keep drinking. Solutions like Gatorade or Pedialyte, which help restore electrolytes lost through vomiting, are great. I've found that Pedialyte freezer pops are a godsend.

Staying seated or walking around a bit after eating is also a good way to prevent heartburn—and don't lie down! When you're upright, gravity helps keep those stomach contents where they belong—down there in your stomach, not rising up into your esophagus. If nature alone isn't doing her job, you can also take Mylanta, Tums, or another antacid. Zantac may be a good antidote to nausea if taken in low, occasional doses (but check with your doctor).

Certain kinds of foods are naturally kinder to an upset stomach. Meals that are rich in complex carbohydrates—whole grains, whole-grain bread—combat nausea. Spicy, greasy foods, on the other hand, tend to promote it. A good rule is to figure out what tastes, smells, or types of food trigger your nausea/vomiting—and then avoid them! Some women keep a daily log, jotting a quick note to themselves whenever they feel sick, as well as noting what they've eaten, when they've cooked, and what foods they've been exposed to. Plotting your symptoms can help you figure out your own triggers.

Many women find that defizzed cola or ginger tea helps to calm an upset stomach. Your doctor may also recommend a high-glucose solution or, in more severe cases, an antinausea medication. Vitamin B_6 in small amounts also seems to be helpful for some women, though there are no scientific studies to support its usefulness.

"Sea bands"—bands that fit around the wrist, bearing down on the acupressure point located there—were invented to combat sea-sickness as a natural alternative to Dramamine (motion-sickness medication); some women find these helpful. There are even "relief bands" that contain electrical devices to stimulate the nerves at the wrist, for acupressure control of nausea and vomiting.

"Pedialyte pops saved my life," recalls Miriam. "They got me through those first three months when it seemed like *nothing* would stay down. Whenever I just couldn't face the thought of food, I'd have one—and I could really feel the difference."

Coping with Nausea/Vomiting—Some Things to Try

- Sea bands/acupressure.
- "Relief bands" that stimulate acupressure points on the wrist by means of electrodes.
- Hypnosis—for relaxation.
- Having someone else prepare meals, empty the litter box, and change your other children's diapers.
- Ginger products, such as ginger ale, ginger tea, pickled ginger, and ginger preserves. The thromboxane synthetase inhibitor in ginger seems to affect testosterone in a way that may help prevent morning sickness. However, there are no long-term studies of ginger's effects on the fetus, so stay away from concentrated ginger capsules.
- Particular foods—your call. Scientists have not yet identified foods that interfere with the natural course of morning sickness, but some women find that potato chips, lemonade, Granny Smith apples, or the smell of lemons helps them control their

nausea. If you experience particular cravings, take advantage of them as soon as possible, before the craving disappears and the "window of opportunity" to nourish yourself is lost.

- High-fluid foods—watermelons and other succulent fruits. These help keep you hydrated.
- Dry crackers and cereal—dry foods generally, early in the morning.
- Ice chips—also good for hydration.
- Ice pops—especially Pedialyte freezer pops.
- Air-conditioning—many women find they feel worse in hot, humid weather.
- Dressing warmly in cold weather—artificial heaters can "dry you out," causing you to lose fluids, which can lead to dehydration and constipation.
- Dill pickles—yes, it's a cliché, but the dill seems to soothe some women's gastrointestinal systems.
- "Mouth rinses" of fresh lemon juice mixed with water—the fresh, citrusy taste can combat that "bad taste in the mouth" feeling that often accompanies nausea, while the lemon scent might mask nauseating odors.
- Hard candies—strong sour or cinnamon-flavored candies can also keep your mouth feeling fresh and clean while blocking the tastes and smells that nauseate you.

Coping with Nausea and Vomiting—Some Things to Avoid

- Things that smell—food, pet products, gas stations, coffeepots, diapers. You might also need to avoid kitchen odors—greasy food, sink drains, and the like. Again, figure out your own triggers—which may change over the course of your pregnancy.
- Sources of "visual vagal stimulation"—that is, visual stimuli that can make you nauseous, such as poor-quality computer screens or jumpy videos.
- Air travel—its charming combination of turbulence, food smells, other people's cologne, and anxiety can all contribute to nausea and vomiting. One of my patients, a frequent traveler, used to

carry a lemon in a resealable plastic bag, so she could sniff it to mask "trigger smells" on long flights.

Coping with Nausea and Vomiting:
Some Medications to Explore with Your Doctor

- Emetrol, also known as phosphorated carbohydrate solution—reduces smooth muscle contractions, but may cause occasional abdominal pain and diarrhea.
- Vitamin B_6, or pyridoxine—helps metabolize carbohydrates, proteins, and fats. Consult with your doctor before you medicate yourself.
- Zantac, or ranitidine—decreases nausea by reducing gastric acid. If you take Zantac, you'll need to take extra B_{12} (check with your doctor) and you may suffer from headaches.

In Extreme Cases . . .

Obviously, most doctors prefer not to prescribe strong medications during pregnancy. Occasionally, though, the mother's and babies' health may be more compromised by vomiting, dehydration, and malnutrition than by the possible side effects of a prescription drug. If yours is one of those extreme cases, your doctor may consider one of the following medications:

- Benadryl, or diphenhydramine—carries the risk of drowsiness, low blood pressure, and other side effects.
- Unisom, or doxylamine succinate—an antihistamine that also tends to sedate.

In the most severe cases, your doctor may prescribe a *Category C* medication—a drug on which animal studies have been done, but no controlled human ones. Possible Category C antinausea drugs include Reglan, or metoclopramide, or Compazine, or prochlorperazine.

What if your nausea and vomiting are pretty much under control—but only because you're living on saltines and ice pops? In that

Fat Is Your Friend

For those of us who have been trying to avoid every extra ounce of fat since our teenage years, the notion that fats and oils can be *good* for a multiple pregnancy comes as quite a radical idea. It's true, though. While you're carrying twins, triplets, or quads, you need to be getting a lot of extra calories from *somewhere,* just to give your body the energy it needs. Moreover, if you're burning up fat during your pregnancy—because you *are* using up lots of extra calories—the by-products of that process, called *ketones,* can actually hurt the fetuses you're carrying.

Many doctors don't understand this—so find a nutritionist who does. It's actually okay for you to be eating ice cream, bacon, cheeseburgers, and all the other things you may have trained yourself to avoid—so enjoy one of the benefits of multiple pregnancy and get some fat-based calories into your system! Just make sure that you're also getting the protein, calcium, and other nutrients that you need.

case, you should consider either regular or high-calorie protein supplements, such as Ensure, Sustecal, or Boost. Many companies will deliver these supplements to you if you are on bed rest, so talk to your doctor or nutritionist about what he or she recommends.

The Right Stuff

The rules for healthy eating during pregnancy aren't all that different from the rules of healthy eating, period. And your needs during a twin pregnancy are pretty similar to those of a woman carrying a singleton—except that you need to take in at least 300 calories more each day.

Here are the two essentials in your multiple-pregnancy diet:

Protein. You should be eating at least four four-ounce servings a day of various types of protein: fish, fowl, red meat, rice and beans, soy

For Vegetarians and Vegans

If you are a vegetarian (no meat) or vegan (no animal products, including eggs and dairy), I urge you to work very closely with your doctor to be sure that you are not compromising your or your babies' health. A regime that may be perfectly healthy for you alone might not work so well for you while you're pregnant—let alone for the twins, triplets, or quads that you're carrying. Some of my patients have added meat, fish, milk, and eggs to their diets while pregnant, then returned to their vegetarian or vegan diets after they finished nursing. If this is unacceptable, work with your doctor and/or a nutritionist.

protein, nuts, and dairy products. Although there's no hard-and-fast rule about it, I think it's a good idea to eat a wide variety of proteins, rather than sticking to a hamburger every lunchtime or restricting yourself to vegetable protein only. Note that I'm recommending several small helpings of protein, which you'll find easier to digest than one or two large servings.

Calcium. You should be drinking four glasses of milk per day—or getting the equivalent of 1,200 mg of calcium in the form of yogurt, cheese, tofu, sardines, salmon, collard greens, broccoli, seaweed, or Lactaid (milk for the lactose-intolerant). For once in your life, you don't have to worry about your cholesterol—it does go up during pregnancy, but your elevated estrogen levels will protect you from atherosclerosis (hardening of the arteries) and other cholesterol-related dangers. So you can even drink whole milk if you like, though skim milk is fine too. The only reason to worry about the fat is if your doctor thinks you're gaining too much weight too fast.

To be on the safe side, when choosing orange juice you might get a brand that includes a calcium supplement. If you get the kind with pulp in it, you're also adding fiber to your diet. If all else fails, you can take a calcium supplement. Tums E-X, for example, can be very helpful for heartburn as well as providing calcium. However, supplements

The Caffeine Controversy

Should you give up your morning coffee or tea or your favorite after-dinner cappuccino? A recent study showed a higher rate of miscarriage when mothers had very high levels of caffeine breakdown products in their blood, such as might be caused by drinking six or more cups of coffee a day. Other studies show that there may be a small increase in the miscarriage rate and a slightly higher risk of low birth weight among women who drink more than one or two cups a day. Some mothers or babies may also be more susceptible to the effects of caffeine than others.

In summary, then, caffeinated coffee or tea in small amounts will probably not produce any lasting harm to you or your babies. If you can, switch to decaf; if you dearly love your caffeinated coffee or tea, keep it down to one cup per day, and make sure to drink plenty of water.

can cause constipation, so it's better to get calcium naturally in your diet. Calcium may also decrease the incidence of hypertension and preeclampsia, conditions for which multiple moms are at higher risk.

Other Nutrients. On general principles, you want to be eating as wide a variety of grains, fruits, and vegetables as you can squeeze into your diet. The broader the range of your diet, the more different nutrients you're taking into your system. Since there's a lot we still don't know about which vitamins and minerals we need to stay healthy, beat the odds by eating some of everything.

Diet Don'ts

I doubt you'll be much surprised by what's on this *Don't* list! Stay away from:

- **Cigarettes.**
- **Recreational drugs.**
- **Advil and aspirin,** unless specifically prescribed for your preg-

nancy (Tylenol is okay in the prescribed amounts, but NSAIDs—nonsteroidal anti-inflammatory drugs, such as aspirin and ibuprofen—can affect fetal circulation).

- **Alcohol.** Alcohol doesn't actually cross the placenta in amounts of less than two ounces—which means that if you're toasting friends at your baby shower, you can probably get away with a few sips of champagne. But since alcohol is such a well-known poison to fetuses, and since it's hard to measure *exactly* what your personal threshold is, why take chances?
- **Caffeine.** Yes, you can probably have one eight-ounce cup of coffee a day, or a few cups of caffeinated tea, or even some hot chocolate or caffeinated cola, if that's your preference. It may increase your metabolism and set your pulse racing, but in small amounts, caffeine probably won't hurt you or your babies.

Some women ask me about NutraSweet and other artificial sweeteners. I'm not crazy about them from a nutritional standpoint—they tend to make you crave sweets more, not less—and it's true that no extensive studies have been done. On the other hand, so many millions of U.S. women rely on NutraSweet and other artificial sweeteners that if such substances *did* cause birth defects, it seems unlikely that we wouldn't have noticed it by now.

Vitamins and Supplements: Keeping You and Your Babies in Top Form

Opinions on vitamins and nutritional supplements vary widely in the medical community these days. Some practitioners recommend them enthusiastically; others—myself included—prefer to err on the side of caution. Here are my best recommendations:

Yes

- **Calcium.** 1,200 mg per day.
- **A basic pregnancy multivitamin.** Prescribed by your physician. (*Don't* take this with a glass of milk, which will interfere with absorbing the nutrients.)

- **Folic acid, or B$_{12}$.** As we said in Chapter 2, ideally you'll start taking this supplement as soon as you conceive, to combat the possibility of spina bifida. You already get 0.4 to 0.8 mg of folic acid in most standard multivitamins, but most women carrying multiples should also be taking an additional 1 mg per fetus each day. Depending on your personal and family history with spina bifida, your doctor may want you to take up to 4 mg a day.
- **Zinc.** A daily supplement of 5 mg may decrease your risk of infection and lower your risk for PROM—premature rupture of the fetal membranes.
- **Fish oil.** Some studies suggest that the fatty acids in cod liver oil can lower the risk of premature labor. While these studies are inconclusive, you might consider taking a daily dose of cod liver gelcaps. Just be sure to get the ones *without* additional A and D.
- **Iron.** In any pregnancy, your blood volume is increased, and with every additional fetus you're carrying, it's increased that much more. All that extra blood volume increases your chances of dilutional anemia (not enough red blood cells for your increased blood volume)—so your doctor may prescribe an iron supplement. Of course, you're already eating lots of green leafy vegetables and other iron-rich foods such as red meat, organ meats, raisins, and dried fruit, right? (Iron-rich fruits and vegetables are especially useful in combating the constipation that meat and iron supplements can cause.)

Iron is particularly important in a multiple pregnancy, since women with twins suffer from anemia almost two and a half times more often than mothers of singletons. Also, multiple moms face a greater risk of hemorrhage, both before and after birth. So keep your iron levels high throughout your pregnancy!

Sometimes a blood count will be low for reasons other than iron deficiency, such as thalassemia, sickle-cell anemia, GPDG deficiency (a shortage of glucose phosphodehydrogenase, an enzyme needed to prevent anemia; common among Sephardic Jews), or a reaction to medication. So if you think you're taking enough iron and your red blood count is still low, make sure your doctor checks your ferritin

Natural Sources of Iron

- Red meats—beef, pork, lamb, or liver
- Chicken and turkey
- Shellfish and sardines
- Tuna and fish
- Iron-fortified cereals
- Enriched breads
- Wheat germ
- Molasses
- Legumes, baked beans
- Turnip and collard greens
- Spinach
- Prunes, prune juice
- Raisins, dried apricots, and peaches
- Strawberries
- Tomato juice
- Eggs

levels, which will tell you if your anemia is caused by iron deficiency or another factor.

By the way, not all iron supplements are created equal. Some actually include substances that can reduce iron absorption. *Ferrous sulfate* is one form of supplement that boosts the iron available to your blood.

Calcium carbonate, magnesium, and zinc, on the other hand, inhibit iron absorption. So if you're routinely taking 30 mg of these supplements per day and you have anemia, try taking 60 mg per day of ferrous iron, in a preparation that includes no additional ingredients that might inhibit absorption. Also, be sure to eat foods rich in vitamin C at any meatless meals you consume (for example, drink orange juice with your veggie burger). Vitamin C helps convert iron into a form more easily absorbed by the human body, so lower quantities of iron go further.

Now here's my list of *no*'s. Please remember that this list is especially

For Maximum Iron Absorption . . .

- Limit or avoid caffeinated drinks at meals—coffee, tea, caffeinated sodas.
- Take your iron supplements separately from your vitamins and calcium supplements.
- Take your supplements one hour before or two hours after eating bran, fiber supplements, dairy products, or eggs.

tailored to pregnant women. Some of these supplements may be perfectly fine when there's no baby involved, but they're apt to cause problems or pose unnecessary risks during pregnancy.

No

- **Vitamin B supplements.** You're already getting all the extra vitamin B you need in your pregnancy multivitamin. Much more B than that (except for the folic acid we've already discussed) is really not a good idea. Too much pyridoxine, or B_6, is known to cause nerve damage—so stay away from high-dose vitamin supplements. (However, in select cases of severe nausea and vomiting, your doctor may advise you to take small doses of B_6.)
- **Vitamin C.** Again, it may be fine to take megadoses of vitamin C if you're *not* pregnant (though I personally am not convinced), but during pregnancy it's not necessary to take more C than you're already getting in your multivitamin. If you're concerned about your C intake, drink orange, grapefruit, or tomato juice and eat plenty of fruit.
- **Other vitamins, nutritional supplements, herbal medicines.** If you feel absolutely committed to a particular supplement or herb, discuss it with your doctor. But remember: Vitamins have a profound impact on the human body, herbs can have potent medicinal effects—and anything that's true for you goes double, triple, or quadruple for the babies you carry. Start your preg-

---

If You're Having Trouble Taking Your Vitamins . . .

- Take two pills in smaller doses, rather than one big pill.
- Time your intake for at least one hour after eating. That's the best time for your system to absorb iron.
- If iron is particularly hard for you to digest, try taking it in liquid form, gelcaps, or new chewables available now.
- Some women digest pills better when they're ground up and taken in applesauce (a chance to baby *yourself* a little before the actual babies come!).

---

nancy with a full and frank discussion in which you tell your physician about *everything* that you are likely to consume. Don't assume that a "natural," herbal, or nutritional product won't affect your baby.

With the recent rise in the popularity of "nutraceuticals," herbal supplements, and natural remedies, pregnant women are more likely to be taking some type of supplement than ever before. Over the past few years, I've seen my patients experiment with ginseng, black cohosh, creatine, androstenedione, and DHEA supplements, among others, and I always advise them to cut out these items during their pregnancy. These remedies are potent—which is why people want to take them—but they aren't regulated, and there are no long-term studies of their effects. When in doubt, use caution—and ask your physician!

8.

Creating Healthy Babies: Medications

❧

Miriam and her husband, Ira, hadn't planned to get pregnant. When they first heard the news, they both had to make several adjustments. I'd been seeing Miriam for several years, so by the time of her first pregnancy visit, we were old friends. I wasn't prepared, though, for how worried she seemed.

"Look, Gila," she told me bluntly. "I've just started taking antidepressants, and they really seem to be helping. And I hate to even think of going through an asthma attack without my inhaler. But now that I'm pregnant, I suppose I'll just have to tough it out."

I was happy to set her straight. Although her doctor might want to adjust her asthma medication and her antidepressant prescription to take account of her pregnancy, she could certainly continue both types of medication. In fact, as far as the asthma medication was concerned, she'd run into problems if she *didn't* keep taking it.

Medications: What You Can Take, Can't Take, Must Take

The best rule for medications is: *Don't assume anything.* Don't assume that any medication is safe to take—but don't assume, either, that you should quit taking all medications the moment you become pregnant. Keep to simple regimens if possible—avoid a polypharmacy!

As with everything else, you should review this subject thoroughly with your doctor. You may also want to do some research of your own. (Take another look at Chapter 2, where we've also discussed medications and offered some suggestions for research on the Internet.) In this chapter, I offer you a basic orientation to help put your doctor's orders and your own research findings in perspective.

DO *Continue to Take*

- **Asthma medication.** Chronically low oxygen levels in the mother can interfere with the fetus's growth. So, as I explained to Miriam, it's bad for the baby if wheezing and other asthma symptoms keep you from getting enough oxygen into your lungs. Asthma medication regimes vary widely, of course, but you'll probably follow the same pattern of medication as before you were pregnant. However, you may require different levels of medication as your pregnancy proceeds. Miriam's asthma actually improved during pregnancy, as it happened, although I've seen other patients' asthma get worse. Either way, it's important to control symptoms and treat upper-respiratory infections aggressively. Make sure your doctor is tailoring your medications to each stage of your pregnancy and to your individual reactions.
- **Antiseizure medications.** It's bad for the babies if you have a seizure—so you will probably need to continue medications that can help you prevent such an occurrence. Let your doctor know that you are planning to conceive, since he or she may need to alter your medications to safer ones before conception and/or alter your dosage to respond to your pregnancy and your ever-expanding volume of blood.
- **Thyroid medication.** Your babies need you to have a healthy, functioning thyroid, so if you've been prescribed medication for a hyper- or hypothyroid condition, do continue to take it. In fact, hyper- or hypothyroidism can cause complications, so make sure you are being monitored regularly, with blood-level

screening. For all pregnant women, measuring basic thyroid function is a good idea.

- **Antidepressants—if necessary.** Although your doctor may wish to switch your prescription, there is probably some kind of antidepressant you can safely take if it's important for you to stay on this medication. Miriam, for example, was taking Prozac, which seems to be pregnancy-safe. Although some studies have shown third-trimester complications, such as increased risk of premature delivery, low birth weight, and poor neonatal adaptation, most studies support the drug's safety during pregnancy. Talk to your doctor about the best antidepressant for you to take, and stay in close touch with your physician and pediatrician if you are breast-feeding.

DO Work with Your Doctor to Find a Substitute For

- **Hypertension medication.** If you've been medicated for high blood pressure, you need to continue some kind of medical regime—but not necessarily the same medication that you took before. Work this out with your doctor as soon as possible. Marsha, for example, had been taking an ACE inhibitor before she got pregnant. During the pregnancy, she switched to Aldomet. After she gave birth, she went back to her ACE inhibitor.
- **Diabetes medication.** Obviously, you'll continue taking insulin and monitor your glucose—but in doses adjusted by your doctor and with even closer surveillance of your sugar levels. If you've been taking other medications for diabetes-related conditions, discuss them with your doctor as well. You will of course be monitoring your glucose levels *very* carefully during pregnancy. (For more on diabetes during pregnancy, see Chapters 13 and 14.)
- **Migraine medication.** Although there are many migraine medications you *can't* take, such as Imitrex, there are some headache remedies you *can* take, such as Tylenol (which many women don't find effective for migraines), Fiorinal (in small doses only), and some beta blockers. Migraine patterns tend to change anyway during pregnancy, so you may find you no longer need your old medication, at least until the babies are born. But if migraine

continues to be a concern, talk to your doctor. There is almost certainly some headache relief that he or she can prescribe. (For more on migraine, see page 107.)

TALK TO YOUR DOCTOR About the Dangers of Taking

- **Lithium.** If you need to keep a bipolar disorder in check or are taking lithium for another condition, talk to your doctor about its use.
- **Accutane.** This antipimple medication is *not* safe during pregnancy.
- **Chloramphenicol, tetracycline, some other antibiotics.** These types of medication are low in side effects if you're *not* pregnant, but they might cause birth defects if you are. Ask your doctor about substitutes.
- **Valproic acid.** You run a 1 to 2 percent risk of your babies developing spina bifida with this medication, which is prescribed as an antiepilepsy drug and as an antidepressant.
- **Dilantin.** This antiepilepsy drug has been shown to cause fetal hydantoin syndrome (facial anomalies) up to 25 percent of the time. However, it's now believed that most other antiepilepsy medications can cause fetal abnormalities—although it's also suspected that the epilepsy itself, rather than the drugs used to treat it, is responsible. Therefore, you should continue to take the safest antiepilepsy medication that's most effective for you, as your doctor closely monitors your pregnancy. You doctor might also suggest that you take 4 mg per day of folic acid, as well as some vitamin K and vitamin D to counteract the possible effects of an antiepileptic drug.

One final caution: Your blood volume increases vastly during a multiple pregnancy, which means that the dosage of virtually *any* medication you're taking will almost certainly have to be adjusted. Moreover, your pregnancy-elevated hormone levels can increase the liver enzymes in your system—enzymes that break down some drugs. Likewise, your increased kidney function might excrete drugs more readily from your system, while antacids that you're taking for nausea, or vomiting itself, can interfere with your absorption of certain drugs. The various ways in which pregnancy can affect your body's relationship to medication is yet another reason to talk to your doctor about medications as early as possible.

Cold and Flu Remedies

I've always felt that these medications are a testament to the American wish for a quick fix. They don't actually shorten your illness, though they may relieve some of your symptoms.

If colds or flu are making you highly uncomfortable, check with your doctor. He or she may have some nonmedicinal suggestions to relieve your discomfort, such as using steam or a vaporizer to unclog your nasal passages, an aromatic rub to ease an aching chest, or extra sleep and time in bed to recover from the exhaustion that colds or flu can bring. (Here is one more time when the apparent discomforts of a multiple pregnancy can be a blessing in disguise: Instead of toughing it out at work using your favorite extra-strength cold medication, you have permission to take to your bed with a detective novel and a hot, soothing drink!)

If you feel that you really must have some kind of medication, check with your doctor. He or she may be able to suggest a mild, single-component cold or flu remedy. Stay away from multicomponent products, such as an antihistamine plus aspirin or a cold remedy that contains cough suppressant and a sleep aid.

Use the same care ingesting "natural" products that you would in taking aspirin or NyQuil. Don't dose yourself with vitamin C or echinacea unless you're under the supervision of someone who knows how these herbs and vitamins might affect the fetuses growing inside you. Remember—anything that's powerful enough to eliminate your symptoms may affect your babies.

Coping with Allergies

My best advice on this topic is to avoid medication by staying away from allergens. But obviously there are limits to this advice: If you live in ragweed country, you can't exactly avoid going outdoors! In that case, you may use Claritin and some antihistamines; again, check with your doctor. Some cough suppressants may also be useful to help you sleep, but do check for alcohol content and find out which ones are pregnancy-safe.

By the way, some of my patients report that acupuncture and Reiki treatments have helped them combat the worst of their allergy symptoms, in some cases quite dramatically. While there are no proven medical benefits to these treatments and I myself remain skeptical, they *are* pregnancy-safe, and they might make you feel better.

What About Antibiotics?

As with many of the other medications I've discussed in this chapter, there's no one simple answer to this question. You don't want to be taking any more medication than you can possibly help—but if you get an infection such as strep throat or a urinary-tract infection, then you *must* take antibiotics to prevent the infection from compromising your pregnancy. There are many safe antibiotics that your doctor might prescribe.

Can You Be Vaccinated?

I've already discussed the question of vaccinations in Chapter 2, where I pointed out that pregnant women can't be vaccinated for German measles, chicken pox, or any other disease whose prevention involves being injected with live attenuated (weakened) vaccines. However, you can have a tetanus shot if you need one, and a flu vaccine is perfectly fine. If you were in the middle of a course of hepatitis vaccines when you got pregnant—there are three altogether—you can finish the series. You shouldn't start a new course, though. For any other questions on vaccines, check with your doctor.

Migraine Treatment and Prevention: Alternatives to Medication

Migraine is an especially exhausting and frustrating type of head pain—and one particularly common to women. The actual headache pain in migraines is caused by an overfull blood vessel in the skull going into spasm. Some women notice that their migraines are preceded by an "aura" lasting 30 to 60 minutes, in which they have vision changes or feel unusually sensitive to light, noise, or other sensations. Migraines themselves can be accompanied by nausea, vomiting, numbness on one side of the face, tingling, changes in vision, or even aphasia (difficulty in saying what one wishes or in comprehending what's being said).

Of the women who suffer from migraine headache before pregnancy, one-third have fewer headaches during pregnancy, one-third have more, and one-third notice no change. The changes in headache patterns seem to be related to hormonal changes, although scientists don't yet understand the relationship completely.

If you do seem to be getting migraines, you may not be able to use the medications that were available to you before pregnancy. Talk to your doctor about pregnancy-safe treatment. You can also learn a great deal from listening to your body to identify particular headache *triggers*. Migraines can be set off by a wide range of causes, including certain foods (hard cheese; red wines; hard liquor; sugar; caffeine; nitrites; and other additives, preservatives, or food dyes); going without food (causing a drop in blood sugar); changes in sleep patterns; weather; bright lights; and emotional stress. Some women find that they're virtually immune to some common migraine triggers while remarkably sensitive to others. Other women notice that they're vulnerable to, say, a dietary trigger when they're feeling tired or stressed, though they seem to be immune at other times. Still other women notice that aerobic exercise—or, during pregnancy, relaxation, deep breathing, and release of stress—helps blunt the power of migraine triggers.

If this problem is of particular concern to you, there are many excellent books on the market that will help you better understand your migraines, avoid your personal migraine triggers, and explore nonmedical ways of preventing and treating migraine headaches.

Dental Work

Your dental hygiene is important during your pregnancy, because any infections in your mouth or gums might eventually affect your babies.

Some Pregnancy-Safe Approaches to Migraine

- **Learn your triggers.** Avoid the foods or situations that set off a migraine. If you can't avoid certain triggers (damp weather, bright lights, noise, stress), respond with deep breathing or some other form of relaxation.
- **Eat regularly and avoid sweets, especially before bedtime.** Falling blood sugar is one of the most common migraine triggers. Some people get headaches from going too long without food; others find that sweet foods bring on a headache because they make the blood sugar rise quickly and then suddenly crash. Your blood sugar falls to its lowest level during the eight or more hours that you're asleep—i.e., not eating—so if you tend to wake up with a headache, try eating some cottage cheese and crackers before you go to sleep. You might also wake up during the night and have a few more crackers or a glass of milk.
- **Exercise—gently.** Migraines are set off by blood vessels constricting too tightly and then opening too quickly in response. Brisk walking and other pregnancy-safe aerobic exercise will help keep your blood vessels open. So will yoga, tai chi, and other types of meditative exercise. (For more on pregnancy-safe exercise, see Chapter 9.)
- **Take advantage of heat and cold.** In the period when you think a migraine might be coming on—after a particularly stressful day or if you're experiencing the "aura"—heat can help relax your body and open your constricted blood vessels. A hot bath, a heating pad, or a heated eye mask are all good ways to take advantage of heat. During the migraine itself, cold helps bring an overly full blood vessel down to its normal size to end your migraine. Ice packs, some ice cubes wrapped in a plastic bag, a washcloth stored in the freezer, or a chilled eye mask can all help you apply cold to your headache pain.
- **Find ways to relax.** Deep breathing, meditation, self-hypnosis, massage, visualization, or any of the other suggestions discussed in Chapter 4 can help release the tension that triggers a migraine. Self-hypnosis and visualization can also be helpful in responding to a headache and easing its pain.
- **Consider biofeedback and acupuncture.** These pregnancy-safe approaches have helped many migraine sufferers. The medical data on these techniques varies widely, but there are several studies suggesting that people who use them get fewer and less-severe migraines.
- **"Talk to your headache."** Some women feel that their migraines are messages that their body is sending itself. If you're getting more headaches than you're comfortable with, try writing in your journal about what's going on for you. Are you doing too much? Doing things you don't enjoy? Are headaches your only way to slow down and rest without feeling guilty? You can write about these issues in a straightforward way, or, for a more playful approach, "ask" your headache what it's telling you and then write the reply from your headache's point of view. You might be surprised what you discover!

Gingivitis might even be a risk factor for premature labor. You'll probably find that your gums are bleeding more than usual because of the increased volume of blood in your body (for more on these changes, see Chapter 10), so it's okay to delay a routine dental cleaning if you like. However, do floss regularly. And if you get a toothache or dental discomfort of any kind, you must go to the dentist.

If your dentist needs to take X rays, that's fine, as long as your abdomen is shielded with a lead apron—protection that your dentist should be offering in any case. If you need a filling, your dentist should avoid Novocain with epinephrine, but a local anesthetic alone is okay. You will probably want to remind your dentist that you're pregnant when you make your appointment.

9.

Creating Healthy Babies:
Exercise, Work, and Rest

⚜

had always wondered when Marsha found the time to exercise. Before she got pregnant, she had an even busier schedule than mine, especially since running her company involved so much overseas travel. She and I were both committed runners, and we often compared notes on how to manage a ten-mile run when you were staying in a strange city on a tight business schedule—or after you've been up all night delivering twins!

I was prepared for Marsha's dismay when I told her that at some point in the pregnancy, the jogging would have to go. But I needn't have worried. With her typical "cover all bases" approach, she had already done a thorough job of researching the kinds of exercise that she *could* enjoy for the next nine months. All she wanted was my opinion on whether yoga or tai chi offered the best supplement to the swimming and walking regimen she had already planned for herself.

When it came to cutting back on her work and travel schedule, though, Marsha was less flexible. "I've spent my life struggling to get here," she said quietly. "Am I supposed to just throw it all away?"

Steering a Middle Course

In this chapter, I'll try to help you steer between two rocky shores. On one side, you hear the siren song of those who insist that you can be Supermom. Even while pregnant with two, three, or even four babies, these voices insist, you should be working, caring for your other children, and getting exercise at pretty much the same level that you did before you got pregnant. Another version of this "Supermom seduction" is the image of the singleton-pregnant mom—maybe even you yourself, in an earlier pregnancy—who pretty much *could* keep up her prepregnancy pace for most of her term.

On the other side, you may be prey to voices that insist you should go right to bed and stay there, to the doomsayers and worriers who anxiously remind you that multiple pregnancies are high-risk. If you don't know any other multiple moms, these voices can be especially frightening.

The truth, in all probability, lies somewhere in between. You probably *will* have to cut back on your busy life, get more rest, and take care of yourself differently. You *may* have to undergo bed rest, for some or all of your pregnancy. Most likely, though, you'll be able to do a lot—if not all—of the things you enjoyed before your pregnancy, stay at work for at least part of your term, and get moderate exercise at something close to the level you've been used to.

The details, of course, will depend on your own individual situation, and you'll have to fine-tune them with your doctor. But in this chapter, I'll give you an overview of what you can expect as far as exercise, work, and physical activity.

Exercise: Feeling Good and Preparing for Childbirth

Exercise is great! It helps keep you physically fit, reduces your level of stress, and improves your chances of an easier pregnancy and a smoother delivery.

On the other hand, if you're pregnant with twins, triplets, or other multiples, you're undergoing a high-risk pregnancy—and exercise may not always be the best policy. The exercise you can do while pregnant is based on the exercise you were doing before pregnancy, as well as on the particular needs of your multiple pregnancy. So have another frank and full discussion with your doctor.

As a general rule, be careful not to get overheated, exhaust yourself, or become dehydrated. Always start with a 10-to-15-minute warm-up period and end with a 10-to-15-minute cooldown. Do *not* stretch vigorously, as your ligaments and joints are more lax during pregnancy.

You probably won't be able to exercise at all if:

- you're at particular risk for preterm labor;
- you've had persistent bleeding during the first trimester;
- your blood pressure is too high;
- your fetuses' growth seems to be restricted.

Generally, though, what you were in shape to do before you got pregnant will be fine.

Jogging is probably the least "pregnancy-friendly" aerobic exercise, since it puts pressure on the cervix and groin muscles. You certainly should not take up jogging during pregnancy, but if, like Marsha, you've been doing it for a while, you may be able to continue during the first trimester. After that, the weight gain and large belly of a multiple pregnancy make it hard—and in some cases, dangerous—to keep running. The American College of Obstetricians and Gynecologists says that you should probably run less than two miles a day, based on studies saying that 1½-mile runs do not seem to adversely affect the fetus. However, these studies all concerned singletons.

If you do run, pay special attention to the terrain. Don't run on hard surfaces, particularly not on concrete or asphalt, and make sure your shoes offer good support. And of course, don't run—or do any other outdoor exercise—if the temperature or humidity is up.

Exercises that are good throughout your pregnancy include *recumbent biking, swimming, yoga,* and *tai chi.* If you're used to *weight training,* you may continue for a while, but no weights of more than five pounds, please. You can increase the number of your repetitions if you're concerned about maintaining muscle tone. *Walking,* using the *treadmill,* and training on the *Stairmaster* are all good pregnancy exercises, so long as you keep a close eye on your pulse.

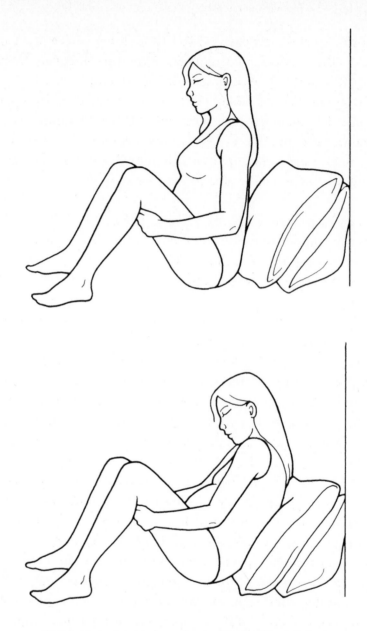

To strengthen abdominal muscles. In sitting position with back support: Knees bent (legs never straight), arms support backs of legs. Breathe in. Breathe out. Pull knees to chest and chin to chest, hold for count of 2, and then relax slowly. Repeat 5–10 times.

FIGURE 1

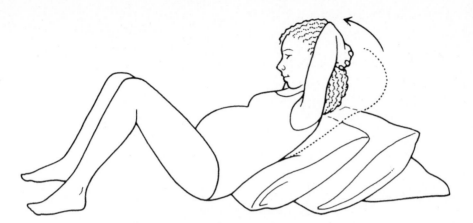

For the first 3 months, you can do these exercises lowering yourself
back on the floor. Do not sit up past the starting position, and
remember to exhale as you sit back.

FIGURE 2

Back pain is common, especially in multiple pregnancies, so choose low-impact exercise. Generally, the rule with exercise is to use your common sense—but err on the side of caution. If you're bleeding or have pain, tell your doctor. To monitor your heart rate—your pulse should not go much above 140—use a heart-rate monitor at your gym or rent one for the duration.

If you are suffering from back pain, a few simple exercises can stretch your muscles and alleviate some discomfort. (See Figures 1 through 4.) However, don't do these exercises lying flat! Use some pillows to support your back.

One final caution: Be careful about exercising at high altitudes. At high altitudes, your blood oxygen levels may decline, so don't exercise at over 8,000 feet, and avoid any kind of exposure to altitudes above 10,000 feet. During your first trimester, you should probably avoid any kind of intense exercise at levels above 6,500 feet, especially if you're anemic or a smoker.

Zoe was struck by the difference between her two singleton pregnancies in her twenties and the twin pregnancy of her thirties. "I'd pretty much stayed in shape since college," she told me, reminding me that she'd been taking various types of aerobics classes at her local Y for as long as she could remember. "But being pregnant with twins knocked me out in a way I just wasn't prepared for."

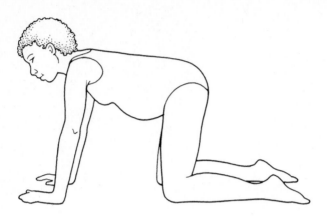

Kneel on floor with your hands directly under your shoulders and keep your back flat.

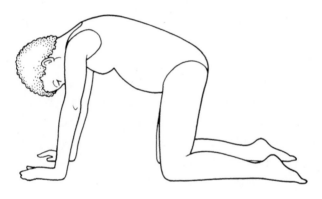

Tighten your abdominal and buttocks muscles and, breathing out, gently tilt your pelvis forward and hump up your back. Hold and then relax. Do not use this exercise to stretch your neck (see Head Rolls, next page). Keep head above heart.

FIGURE 3

Sarah had watched her two sisters go through five pregnancies between them. While neither of her siblings was a world-class athlete, Sarah noticed that each of them had made a point of going for a brisk walk each day, and her older sister had done laps three times a week at her local swim club. "I thought I'd take up swimming too," Sarah told me. "But I was lucky if I could do five laps without collapsing. It certainly made me wish I'd gotten into better shape *before* I got pregnant."

Natalie, on the other hand, breezed through her twin pregnancy with a regular routine of walking, swimming, and yoga, much like the regime Marsha eventually worked out for herself. My own pregnancy experience was much like theirs—I was able to bicycle through my first trimester and to do regular laps at our local pool after that.

Swimming is terrific during pregnancy, by the way, because your ever-growing body makes you more buoyant in the water, and the ex-

FIGURE 4

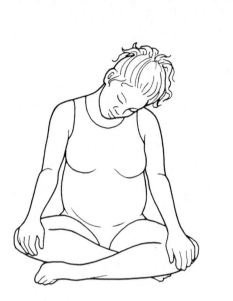

To relieve tension and
increase suppleness.

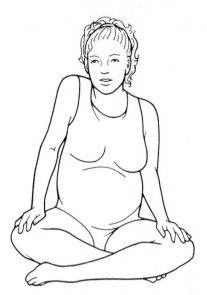

Do head and shoulder rolls
in a circle. Roll head side,
forward, and side.
Do *not* roll back.

ercise feels easier. Studies also show that swimming increases your
urine output and reduces edema (swelling). It's also easier to keep
your temperature stable in the water, as opposed to on-land exercise.
Likewise, your heart rate is usually lower after swimming than after
running or some other on-land exertion. Swimming places less strain
on your uterus than other kinds of exercise and is good for your blood
flow. And, I have to say, when you're carrying around 30, 40, or 50 extra pounds, it feels great to feel *light* in the water!

My point is that every woman is different—and so is every pregnancy. If you've been pregnant before or have known other pregnant
women, you may be struck by the difference between what can be
done during a singleton pregnancy and what can be done by you, the
mother of twins, triplets, or higher-order multiples. In all likelihood,
you can—and should—do some kind of physical activity, but you may
need to limit it if complications develop. After all, your *main* fitness
goal is to complete your pregnancy in good health—with two or
more healthy babies. Remember, multiple pregnancy is in itself a cardiovascular challenge!

Working Things Out at Work

For most of us, work is a highly charged issue. It's not only the place where we spend more hours than anywhere else, it's also an important part of our identities, a key social network—and, almost certainly, a major component of our family financial resources. If we're in a profession or at a managerial level that is in any way unusual for a woman, we're especially loath to do anything to suggest that we can't cut it or that we need special treatment of any kind. And if we have a business of our own, whether as a self-employed freelancer or as the CEO of a small company, the pressure to keep performing at prepregnancy levels can be enormous.

To add to the pressure, many multiple moms get pregnant later in life, at the height of their careers or at a point where they're just starting to feel successful. Marsha wasn't the only one of my patients who was distressed at the changes required by her multiple pregnancy. "I'm finally coming into my own," 39-year-old Sarah told me when I explained the special needs of her triplet pregnancy. "How can I cut back now?"

On the other hand, *because* work is so important, emotionally and financially, it may also be one of the most demanding arenas in our lives. And, as such, it may be a place where we need to pull back, at least for a time, while coping with the demands of a multiple pregnancy.

I myself was lucky: I *was* able to keep working. I was in my first year of practice when I got pregnant with my twins, and my then only daughter was three. Night after night, I dragged myself out of bed to attend other women who were giving birth. I vividly recall struggling with the nausea of the first trimester and trying to keep my surgical scrubs from slipping off my newly huge body as my pregnancy progressed. After one delivery, a husband called his mom with the good news and exclaimed, "The delivering obstetrician was bigger than Kate!"

Yet I did a good job caring for my patients and supporting my colleagues in private practice. I delivered babies until 36 weeks and worked until 38 weeks—and my twins were born at 40 weeks at good, healthy weights. Six weeks after delivery, I flew to Chicago to take the most important test of my career, the specialty exam for my certification as an ob/gyn. Despite my exhaustion, I passed with flying colors—and I've been working ever since, through a third pregnancy and a fourth child.

The French Experience

The French have been studying women, work, and pregnancy for many years now, primarily with the goal of developing a national work-leave policy for pregnant women. One landmark French study, conducted in 1984, found that there *was* a significant relationship between exhausting work and premature birth. Of the 3,437 pregnancies studied, 1,928 involved working mothers, subject to five main sources of fatigue:

1. standing more than three hours a day;
2. working on industrial machines;
3. continuous or frequent physical exertion;
4. the mental stress involved in performing repetitive tasks;
5. noisy, cold, wet, or "chemically affected" environments.

Women who rated high on the fatigue scale were far more likely to deliver prematurely. Only about 2 percent of mothers with no fatigue indicators had premature births, whereas over 11 percent of women with all five indicators delivered before term.

Many other French studies have continued to support the idea that cutting back on work is good for many pregnant women, particularly those with physically demanding jobs. In 1989–1991, for example, a much smaller study was conducted of 546 mothers who were pregnant with twins in a western suburb of Paris. These women were told to reduce their physical effort beginning at 22.8 weeks, with work leave prescribed for those who were employed outside the home. Only 5.4 percent of these women's twins were delivered before 32 weeks, while in the United States, in 1987, more than twice as many twin deliveries—11 percent—took place before 32 weeks. This study was criticized for not having a control group—a group of French women who *didn't* cut back on work—and of course, the U.S. and French mothers are not directly comparable. However, a recent U.S. study also found a higher rate of second-trimester hospital and emergency-room visits in women who reported a lot of fatigue and who had to manage both job and home responsibilities.

I include my own story to show that working straight through *is* sometimes possible. Still, for some women, that course is neither possible nor desirable. In fact, the whole topic of how the mother's work affects the fetus is marked by conflicting studies and varied opinions. Some research has found a higher incidence of premature labor (but not premature birth) among working mothers, as well as a decreased birth weight among the infants who were finally born. A prototype of long hours, physical exertion, and fatigue is, of course, the medical residency, and some studies conducted in the 1980s showed that pregnant medical residents did indeed give birth to children with lower birth weights while suffering from increased rates of maternal hypertension. However, not all studies agreed—and certainly my own personal experience did not bear out these conclusions.

On the other hand, if you've had a history of preterm labor or have an incompetent cervix, you're already at risk for preterm labor and should be extra careful. Women in this category may indeed need to consider taking a work leave or cutting back in some other way. Likewise, if your job involves prolonged standing, heavy lifting, vibrations, or exposure to toxins, you may be putting yourself and your babies at risk. Standing for long hours seems to have particularly adverse effects, because it pulls your heavy, pregnant uterus deep into your pelvis and blocks the return of blood from your legs to your heart. This can cause uterine contractions and, possibly, preterm labor.

"Do I Need to Stay in Bed?"

There are two types of bed rest associated with multiple pregnancies: *prophylactic bed rest,* or bed rest used as a general preventive measure; and bed rest *prescribed in response to a specific condition,* generally to prevent preterm labor.

For years, many doctors routinely prescribed prophylactic bed rest in the hospital to the pregnant mothers of twins, triplets, and other higher-order multiples. In my own experience—both as a doctor and as the mother of twins—there's no need for such extreme measures, and a vast body of literature supports this opinion. Study after study has found that hospital bed rest as a *general* preventive measure doesn't improve the outcomes of multiple pregnancies. In fact, prolonged bed

The Not-So-Friendly Skies

Travel is particularly stressful for the woman who's carrying twins, triplets, or quads. Even nonpregnant bodies are working harder at higher altitudes, as several studies of flight attendants have shown. Other studies have revealed that flying can actually decrease a pregnant woman's oxygen level by 25 percent and increase her blood pressure during the time spent at cruising altitude. If a passenger suffers from flight anxiety, her blood pressure goes up even more.

If business travel is a big part of your job, maybe you can work out an alternative arrangement for a few months. Again, what may have been possible for a singleton mother might not be an option for a multiple mom.

If you must travel, try to follow these guidelines:

- Don't carry your own luggage. *Always* get someone else to do it for you. The stress of carrying combined with the fatigue of traveling can pose serious risks to your pregnancy. If you're lugging a laptop and a briefcase full of work, they count as luggage, so yes—find an assistant, skycap, or trustworthy stranger to help you carry your belongings onto the plane.
- Try to eat well. Unless there are some unusual airports on your route, this probably means packing your own food to take with you.
- Drink plenty of water. Plane travel can dry you out under the best of circumstances—and dehydration can increase the risk of uterine contractions. Carry a large, empty water bottle with you onto the plane (anything else will be too heavy), and politely ask the flight attendant to fill it for you—perhaps twice.
- Practice some relaxation and breathing exercises to keep yourself from getting too tense or stressed out. (See Chapter 4 for some suggestions.)
- During a flight of more than two hours, get up, walk around, and stretch to keep the circulation going in your legs. You might request an aisle seat to make this movement easier. I once saw a pregnant woman sitting in the bulkhead seat, her swollen legs resting on an inflatable ottoman that she'd brought along.

rest may cause problems of its own, such as deep venous thrombophlebitis (blood clots), as well as poor muscle tone, which contributes to exhaustion during and after labor.

When Bed Rest Is Prescribed

Sometimes bed rest—usually at home, occasionally in the hospital—*is* an appropriate response to a *specific* problem. If you've had signs of preterm labor, pelvic exams that indicate cervical change, or contractions, then home bed rest will probably be the first step in your treatment.

If you *do* have to stay in bed, take this order *very* seriously. Bed rest doesn't mean staying in bed for an hour, getting up to get a box of photos out of your closet, and then climbing back into bed to work on your photo album. It means *staying in bed.* Let someone else bring you the photos. If you have toddlers at home, they'll quickly learn to climb into bed with Mom for a bedtime story; if you have older children, they may actually enjoy having you as a "captive audience" to whom they can bring snacks, special get-well cards, and stories of their day.

Telling someone to spend every single minute of the day in bed is easier said than done—but yours is a very unusual pregnancy, as you've already realized. If your doctor has prescribed bed rest, it's because he or she is concerned about the possibility of preterm labor. Keep your babies inside your womb as long as possible by staying in bed yourself!

However, mothers of multiples *do* need to rest more than other pregnant women. Remember, your number-one goal as a multiple mom is to prevent preterm labor and keep your babies growing healthily inside you. You can work toward this goal by getting more rest, putting your feet up for a couple of hours each day, and, possibly, cutting back on the physical activities of your daily life.

When the modern women's movement first began, a popular slogan was the notion of "having it all." As Marsha faced the complications in her pregnancy—including two weeks of bed rest—she came up with a powerful response. "You *can* have it all," she told me the day she took her healthy twin boys home from the hospital. "Just not all at the same time." Finding a way to juggle the demands of work and children will be an ever-changing but always-present part of your life as a parent.

10.

What's Happening to Your Body?: The First Trimester

As you pass through the various stages of pregnancy, your body and your babies' bodies will grow and change. In this chapter and the next two, I'll give you an overview of what you might expect and the information you need.

Starting Your Pregnancy

When Sarah and her partner, Philip, found that Sarah was pregnant, it came as a wonderful surprise. Sarah was 39, and the two of them had been together for only two years. Although they had both always wanted children, the time had never been right before. Given Sarah's age, they hadn't even been sure that they *could* have a child together.

On top of the dramatic news of Sarah's pregnancy came the even more surprising revelation that she was carrying triplets. Although both Sarah and Philip welcomed the idea of an "instant family," they were overwhelmed by the suddenness of this change in their life together, as well as concerned about the dangers to Sarah's health and the very real question of whether all three triplets would survive.

"Given everything, we decided to keep the news to ourselves until at least the fourth or fifth month," Sarah explains. "Of course, given how soon I was likely to start showing, we weren't sure we *could* keep it a secret. But our friends hadn't even known we were trying to get pregnant—and we didn't want anyone to be disappointed. We especially didn't want people to expect triplets and then have to explain that we were only having one or two babies."

"Frankly, we both went a little nuts for a while," Miriam says, recalling how she and her husband, Ira, reacted to the news of her twin pregnancy. "It wasn't at all what we expected, and we just didn't want anyone else's input until we got ourselves sorted out. We knew our families would be thrilled—and they were—but we also knew they'd be worried—and they were! I in particular wanted to know just what my medical risks and options were before my mother and Ira's mother had the chance to ask me even a single question."

Natalie, on the other hand, couldn't wait to share the news of her twin pregnancy with her family and friends. "I wanted to shout it from the rooftops!" she says, obviously enjoying what is still a thrilling memory. "I'd wanted twins all my life, and now I had them! I felt so special. I don't think I could have kept it secret if I'd wanted to."

Like most multiple moms, you may find this first trimester a dramatic time, as you make the transition from not-pregnant to pregnant. If it's your first pregnancy, you may feel you don't know what to expect. If you've been pregnant before, you may think you *do* know what to expect—and still run into a few surprises. This is a time for going slowly, for working with your doctor to discover what kind of challenges you may face, for building strong ties with your partner as the two of you embark on this new journey. Like Sarah and Philip, and Miriam and Ira, many couples choose to keep the pregnancy private during this trimester, until the health of the babies is well-established.

How Your Body Is Changing

One of the major changes your body will begin is to increase blood volume. This change occurs in any pregnancy but is especially apparent in a multiple pregnancy, as your blood now nourishes you and at least two other beings. You'll need to drink lots of fluids to maintain this increased volume, and you'll also need plenty of iron to guard against anemia: The number of red blood cells that was sufficient for your prepregnancy body just won't be enough for your new, expanded blood volume. (See Figure 1.)

"I couldn't believe how much iron I seemed to crave," Zoe recalls. "I hate to keep comparing everything to my first two pregnancies, but it's hard not to. I was eating plenty of meat and greens then too—but this time I felt like I was living on steak and spinach."

You'll also begin gaining weight, partly from this new, increased amount of blood, partly from the babies themselves, partly from the placenta and the other material you're carrying. The rate and timing of weight gain can vary dramatically: Although many multiple moms begin gaining weight and showing far earlier than their singleton-bearing sisters, many others actually lose weight during the first trimester, as they may also experience far more nausea and vomiting than singleton moms. I myself actually lost ten pounds in my first trimester pregnant with my twins—and I assure you, I never spontaneously lost ten pounds at any other time in my life! (I wish I'd used high-protein/high-calorie nutritional supplements at that time—I certainly prescribe them now!)

Finally, the hormonal changes that go with pregnancy will begin to make themselves felt in this trimester. As with singleton pregnancies, these changes tend to have different effects at different times, often producing overwhelming fatigue in the first trimester, generally followed by a sense of energy and well-being in the second trimester. "I was all over the place," Miriam recalls. "One minute I'd be my usual busy self; the next minute I'd sink down into a chair and have to fight to keep from crying. I'm sure some of it was the simple fact of being pregnant—and with twins! But it also felt like an exaggerated version of PMS."

Like Miriam, the emotional changes you undergo in response to the pregnancy may well be colored by your hormonal ups and downs, so this is a time to be patient with yourself and to ask others to be patient with you, as you get used to the new contours, moods, and sensations of your multiply-pregnant body.

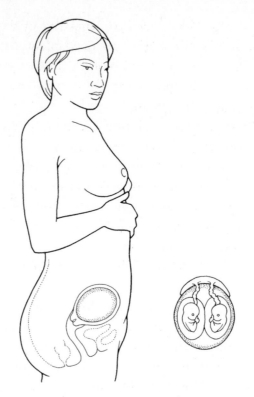

Figure 1. The First Trimester

What You May Notice

- **Fatigue.** "Tiredness," which you've probably felt before, can be addressed with a few nights' sleep or a restful weekend. Pregnancy-related fatigue can be far more draining, since it reflects the great increase in progesterone that marks this stage of pregnancy. (If you've ever felt fatigued just before your menstrual period, this stage of fatigue is hormonally similar.) In my experience, the sudden, sharp, and overwhelming fatigue of a first-trimester multiple pregnancy is always surprising, and often hard to deal with. Sleep, good nutrition, and moderate exercise can all help—but also, most likely, you'll need to slow down. Most pregnant women feel a surge of energy in their second trimester, but it tends to be less dramatic for multiple moms.

- **Increased appetite.** This extra hunger may be especially marked early on in multiple pregnancies—or you may instead experience increased nausea (see below). If you do feel extra hungry during your first trimester, you'll probably notice it sometime between Week 4 and Week 6. Whether your hunger begins then or later, however, you will feel it eventually—and it's likely to continue throughout your pregnancy. "For me, it was weird," Natalie recalls, "because on the one hand, I couldn't stand to eat the kinds of foods I usually like—my diet got real bland, real fast. But on the other hand, I was starving *all the time.* I got real friendly with rice cakes, which had always tasted like Styrofoam to me before—and since. But those first few weeks, especially, they became my favorite food."

- **Nausea, vomiting, a heightened sense of smell.** As we've seen, pregnancy-related hormones decrease the *motility* (ability to move) of your stomach, making it harder for your stomach to fully empty itself. The leftover digested matter can collect stomach acid and make you feel nauseous. Meanwhile, hormonal changes affecting the nervous system can sharpen your sense of smell in unexpected ways—and cause you to feel repulsed or nauseated by odors that you either liked or didn't notice before. ("We had just bought a new car," Jeannette confides, "and the new-car smell, which I'd always loved, suddenly made me want to throw up.") You might also find yourself craving carbohydrates, both to satisfy your hunger and to take the edge off your nausea. Go ahead and eat—just try to stick to whole grains. For more on how to cope with nausea and vomiting—which are usually more intense in multiple pregnancies—see Chapter 7.

- **Heartburn and indigestion.** These reactions, too, are usually more intense in multiple pregnancies. In Chapter 7, we saw how hormones also decrease the muscle tone of your lower esophageal sphincter—the ring-shaped muscle that joins your esophagus to your stomach. Pregnancy-related pressure on your abdomen may push some of your stomach contents—leftover food mixed with digestive acids—back up into the esophagus, and your less efficient sphincter relaxes and lets these acids through. The result:

heartburn and indigestion. For more on this syndrome and how to cope with it, see Chapter 7.

- **Food cravings and taste changes.** This is one of the many times during pregnancy that it pays to listen to your body. You probably *won't* crave the legendary pickles and ice cream—but you might well be hungry for spinach, steak, or other iron-rich foods to combat the mild anemia common in many pregnancies. As your blood volume increases, your body may have trouble making enough extra red blood cells to keep up, so if you do find yourself longing for red meat, leafy green vegetables, and other sources of iron, follow those cravings! And if you've got a yen for foods that are less easily explained, give in to your wishes: At best, you're craving a necessary nutrient; at worst, you just "feel like it." (My fellow residents always knew when I was pregnant because I would invariably order hot sauerkraut with lunch—a food I never touched at any other time!)

- **Constipation.** Pregnant women are prone to this condition—and mothers of multiples even more so. Partly that's because you're bigger, so there's more pressure on your digestive organs. But mothers of twins and other multiples report problems fairly early in the pregnancy, before they've gained much weight, so clearly, pregnancy-related hormones are also involved. Just as your stomach has less motility, so does your intestinal tract, which means that matter moves more slowly through your colon. Meanwhile, your pregnant body is absorbing more water than usual from your stool, and the remaining solids are harder. In Chapter 7, we talked about some ways of avoiding constipation: drink more fluids and eat foods rich in fiber. Moderate exercise helps too. Remember that iron supplements—contained in all prenatal multivitamins—increase the likelihood of constipation, so you may want to add a high-fiber supplement or bulk-forming agent such as Citrucel. Sarah found another solution: prunes in hot water.

- **Dry mouth.** When you're pregnant, you need extra water to support your vastly increased blood volume and all the extra fluids in your breasts, uterus, and elsewhere in your body. The more babies you're carrying, the more fluid—so if you're not drinking enough water to support your pregnancy, you may experience dry mouth.

- **Extra saliva.** On the other hand, if your stomach is irritated, you may not be swallowing as often as you usually do. In that case, you may notice *extra* saliva filling up your mouth. *Ptyalism,* or excess salivation, is a common pregnancy complaint.

- **More frequent urination.** Your bladder is under pressure from your uterus, so it can't hold as much urine. It gets full much more quickly, even at the beginning of your pregnancy, so you have to empty it more often. Also, the same hormonal changes that are relaxing your sphincter and stomach muscles are relaxing your bladder muscles, so you're likely to experience more reflux—that is, your urine may "back up" inside your bladder and flow in the other direction. This makes you more prone to urinary-tract infections (UTIs), so be on the lookout for telltale symptoms:

➢ ALERT: If you notice any burning or pain when you urinate, blood in your urine, pain in your flanks or lower back, or fever along with any of these symptoms, call your doctor right away. You may have a urinary-tract infection, which, especially during pregnancy, may put you at increased risk of kidney infection. That's because the hormones of pregnancy can affect your ureters (the tubes that connect the urinary tract and the kidneys), allowing bacteria to pass from your urinary tract into your kidneys. Of course, sometimes the classic symptoms of burning, frequent urination, and urgent urination may be different. Your practitioner will err on the side of taking a culture of your urine if you're experiencing even the vaguest symptoms of a UTI. UTIs need to be treated with antibiotics during pregnancy.

➢ ALERT: If you notice fever with chills and lower back pain, or blood in your urine, tell your doctor right away, as these are common symptoms of kidney infection. If you do have such an infection, your doctor will probably prescribe intravenous antibiotics and, possibly, hospitalization.

- **Stuffiness.** Since all your mucous membranes are receiving a larger supply of blood, your nasal membranes may swell and secrete extra mucus. Stay away from chemical nasal inhalers, which, when used over time, can produce long-term changes in the tissues that line your nose. Steam inhalers are better, or normal saline drops. (You can save them for when your babies have stuffy noses that they're too little to sneeze clear!) If stuffiness is a chronic problem, you might want to get a humidifier or, for a low-tech approach, place a pot of water on every radiator. ("I put a little Vicks VapoRub under my nose," Natalie recalls. "The menthol fumes seemed to clear me right out.")

- **Nosebleeds.** The little capillaries in your nasal passages are also swelling with blood, and they may simply rupture and bleed.
➢ ALERT: If you're getting bloody noses fairly often, have a yellowish discharge from your nose, or have either symptom plus fever, tell your doctor. Likewise, if you can't stop the bleeding, let your doctor know. He or she may have to cauterize the area.

- **Swollen and/or bleeding gums.** Your gums may swell during pregnancy, which makes them more likely to bleed. Floss and brush gently but consistently, and do attend to toothaches!

- **Hemorrhoids.** This annoying condition gets worse in pregnancy—once again because of the increase in your blood volume, which causes the middle hemorrhoidal veins to dilate. Some 80 percent of women carrying twins report hemorrhoids by the time they reach term. Uncomfortable as this condition is, it's only a real problem if you are bleeding heavily, in which case your doctor may prescribe cortisone enemas or suppositories. (For more on coping with hemorrhoids, see page 133.)

- **Breathlessness,** also known as *dyspnea.* This is the feeling that you can't quite catch your breath or that amidst regular breathing you feel the need to sigh deeply. This condition is common to some 70 percent of all pregnant women, and despite many of my patients' fears, it has nothing to do with being a couch potato. In even the most physically fit woman, the rib cage expands during pregnancy, requiring a larger volume of air to be filled. In a multiple pregnancy, your rib cage expands rather dramatically during the first trimester, in preparation for the extra uterine growth of the second and third trimesters. Thus, you may need to breathe more deeply in order to fill up your lungs. (Toward the end of your pregnancy, you may experience shortness of breath for another reason: Your expanding uterus is pushing on your diaphragm.)

- **Elevated heart rate.** You might notice your heart beating faster while finding yourself more aware of your pulse than you were before. That's because, as we've seen, the volume of your blood is increasing rapidly—you will contain one and a half times your normal volume by the end of your pregnancy—even as pregnancy-related hormones are lowering your blood pressure. As a result, your heart has to work harder and beat faster to keep this extra blood moving through your body without losing blood pressure.

- **Breast tenderness and changes in appearance.** For some women, this is the first sign that they are in fact pregnant. You'll probably notice both tenderness and swelling, with an especially marked increase in your first trimester. By the time your pregnancy is over, you may have gained as many as three cup sizes. ("I'd always been flat-chested," Jeannette says, "so this was one part of pregnancy that I really loved. I felt like an earth goddess." Miriam, on the other hand, says, "I couldn't *believe* how big I got—it was so uncomfortable! Either my bras weren't supportive enough, or they were way too binding.") You may also notice that the veins in your breasts seem more prominent, especially if you're fair-skinned. Again, that's because of increased blood volume, which makes the veins swell. Some women notice that their nipples and areolae (the areas around the nipples) are more darkly colored. It's also common to have some clear fluid leaking from the breast.

➤ ALERT: If you find one particular area of swelling—that is, *localized* swelling—or a lump or nodule anywhere in your breast, tell your doctor right away. Breast cancer can develop in pregnancy as well as at other times, so it pays to stay alert. Likewise, tell your doctor if your nipples ever discharge blood.

- **Changes in sexual feelings.** Read through the pregnancy-related changes on this list—heartburn, fatigue, tender breasts—and then try to imagine how you could *not* experience at least *some* changes in your sexual responses during your pregnancy! Not surprisingly, many women experience a decrease in sexual interest during their pregnancy, either because of hormonal changes or because the experience of pregnancy is so tiring that by 8:00 P.M., the mere thought of having sex seems as remote as Mars. Other women, however, experience increased libido, while still others go through fluctuating sexual responses. For a fuller discussion of sexuality and pregnancy, see Chapter 4.

- **Sensitive skin.** The famous "glow" of pregnancy is more than just the joy of expectant motherhood—it's an actual biological change. As your blood volume increases, extra blood is pumped nearer your skin's surface—and suddenly you look radiant. On the other hand, you're more susceptible to sunburn, so don't stay out in the sun too long, and use a sunscreen (I suggest one with a moisturizer). Your skin may be sensitive in other ways too, so this is probably not the time to experiment with new skin-care products or makeup.

- **Stretch marks.** As your uterus and breasts get larger, the collagen in your skin separates—and you get stretch marks. Good lifelong nutrition seems to work against stretch marks, and women whose skin has more pigment find that their marks are less noticeable. The marks do tend to fade after pregnancy—but they never disappear completely. Try to think of them as a badge of honor, or at least try to accept them as part of the passage into (multiple) motherhood. Other visible marks of pregnancy include skin tags—small brown growths—and linea nigra, literally a "black line" (actually, a dark line) that extends below the belly button. Women with more melanin in their skins tend to have darker lines. These lines tend to fade after pregnancy is over.

➤ ALERT: If you notice a skin tag that is unusually large, of irregular shape, or bleeding, tell your doctor.

- **Mood changes.** It would be pretty remarkable if the hormones that are making you tired and nauseous while relaxing your stomach, bladder, and ureters did not *also* bring mood changes in their wake. If you experienced mood swings or intense feelings during your premenstrual time, you may have some inkling of what pregnancy-related mood changes might feel like. Of course, as with any emotional reaction, it's always difficult to sort out what's a reasonable response to your situation and what's hormonally induced or heightened. Be aware that many women feel anxious, weepy, or angry during this trimester, before enjoying a period of relative calm, serenity, even bliss, in the second three months of their pregnancy.

Tips for Coping

- If you're annoyed by hemorrhoids, your doctor will probably recommend an over-the-counter antihemorrhoid medication, such as Preparation H, or prescription suppositories or enemas. A cold pack applied to the rectal area, a sitz bath for 15 to 20 minutes a day, and keeping yourself well-hydrated should all help ease this condition.
- To combat constipation, try a high-fiber diet—lots of fruits, vegetables, and complex carbohydrates. Drinking plenty of water also makes a huge difference. As we've seen, iron—which you may be taking as a supplement and should certainly be getting in your diet—actually encourages constipation, so you could be subject to something of a vicious cycle. Citrucel, psyllium, unprocessed bran, and other bulk-forming agents may be able to help you break the cycle and calm your digestive system.
- Find some comfortable bras! You probably won't want the underwire kind: brassieres with straps that go across both back and shoulders are far more comfortable. Some women like sports bras for their comfort and support, but as your pregnancy proceeds, these may seem too restrictive. You can probably find the bras you want in most department stores, which often sell pregnancy brassieres that convert to nursing bras. ("I finally *did* find the perfect bra halfway through my eighth month," Miriam recalls. "I have it saved in a special place just in case I ever get pregnant again—although, unless it's twins, I probably won't get quite so big!")
- Learn the pregnancy-safe way to use a seat belt. The proper fastening of a seat belt around your extra-large uterus is of utmost importance to protecting you and your unborn children. Auto accidents account for about half of the trauma cases that complicate 6 to 7 percent of all pregnancies. Most of the time, this is a minor

problem—but 1 to 3 percent of all minor traumas end in the loss of a fetus. New studies suggest that pregnant women should not buckle the lap belt over their uterus. Rather, the lap belt should be placed as low as possible below the pregnant "bulge," while the shoulder belt should be put on the side of the pregnant abdomen, between your breasts and over the center of your clavicle (collarbone).

- Prepare to take it easy! I tell my patients to cut out any extra social obligations and concentrate on just getting through the day. For most multiple moms, if they can manage the commute, the day at work, and the absolutely necessary household chores (especially if there are children at home), they've had a good day. Now is not the time to start that new book club or plan a neighborhood fund-raiser. You might not even feel like running out for a night of dinner, theater, and late-night ice cream. Cut back wherever you can—and, equally important, adjust your expectations to fit your new reality. Find ways of feeling *successful* as you manage your new, demanding role as a multiply-pregnant mom.

What Your Monthly Doctor's Visits Will Include

Diagnostic Visit

- **Blood-pressure test.**
- **Examination of your skin.** The skin is your largest organ, and its condition gives the doctor lots of insight into *your* condition. Very dry skin could indicate that you have hypothyroidism (an underactive thyroid). Skin lesions can be evidence of infection. High estrogen levels contribute to that pregnancy "glow," but they also cause veins in your legs and elsewhere to swell, as well as adding a reddish tone to your palms and the heels of your hands. Some women develop "the mask of pregnancy": a redness or additional pigmentation on the bridge of the nose, extending beneath the eyes. This will fade after your babies are born.
- **Examination of your breasts.** Your doctor will look closely at your skin, nipples, and areolae (the areas around the nipples), and

palpate (feel) your breasts for any masses. He or she will also check your axilla (armpit) for any nodes or masses.

• **Pelvic exam.** Both your external genitalia and your vagina will be checked for lesions and to make sure the skin looks normal. Your doctor will also palpate the uterus, examine your tubes and ovaries, and check your cervix, to ensure that there are no problems there.

• **Assessment of your abdomen.** Your doctor will check for the presence of hernias or a *diastasis recti* (the separation of the abdominal wall muscles), as well as check out the size of your uterus, liver, and spleen.

• **Examination of your neck.** Your doctor will palpate your neck to see if there's an enlargement caused by thyroid or any other unusual masses.

• **Evaluation of your back.** If you have scoliosis (curvature of the spine) or arthritis, your doctor needs to know as soon as possible, since it may affect your choices about how to deliver your babies.

• **Assessment of your musculoskeletal system.** Your doctor will want to know whether your arms and legs can move freely and whether you have any history of trauma. A check of your reflexes will also help him or her better understand your nervous system.

• **Scrutiny of your lungs and heart.** Your doctor needs a baseline for both these important organs so that if you develop shortness of breath, he or she can determine how serious the problem is. Your doctor will also want to be sure that your heart is normal in size, location, and rhythm, and to know whether you have a heart murmur or any other abnormality that might affect pregnancy or delivery. If you have been seeing this doctor for some time, he or she may not need to perform this exam, as the baseline data is already available.

• **Urine sample.** Your doctor will be checking your urine every month for signs of vaginal or urinary-tract infections, or for protein and excess glucose.

• **Pap smear.** This test will reveal any abnormal or precancerous cell growth on your cervix.

- **Vaginal cultures.** These exams help rule out gonorrhea, chlamydia, or bacterial vaginosis. If you do suffer from one or more of these conditions, you and your doctor will have to discuss the treatment and follow-up.
- **Blood tests.** Among other procedures, you'll have a test for syphilis; the rubella titer to see if you're immune to rubella (German measles); tests for hepatitis B and HIV; a complete blood count (CBC) to make sure you don't have anemia; and an evaluation of your blood type, Rh factor, and presence of irregular antibodies. If your and your babies' blood is not compatible, your pregnancy will be more closely monitored (see Chapter 13).
- **Tuberculosis test.** As a routine precaution, your doctor will probably be testing you for TB.
- **Vaccines.** Your doctor may vaccinate you with Pneumovax against *Streptococcus pneumoniae,* a form of pneumonia, and with the influenza vaccine if you're pregnant during flu season (October 1 to March 31).
- **Human chorionic gonadotropin (hCG) assessment.** This hormone in the blood and urine is what's measured in a home pregnancy test—it's also known as the "pregnancy hormone." A higher than normal level of hCG might indicate twins, triplets, or quads.
- **Monitoring progesterone levels.** Your doctor may want to keep track of this aspect of your hormonal activity if you've had ovulation induction, IVF, or a history of miscarriage.

Your Second and Third Months

- **Blood test for hemoglobin.** If your doctor is concerned about anemia, he or she may test your hemoglobin (red blood cell) levels.
- **Assessment of weight gain.**
- **Blood-pressure test.**
- **Evaluation of pulse and respiratory rates.**
- **Examination of heart and lungs.**
- **External palpation of the uterus.**
- **Physical assessment of your breasts.**

- Urine sample—screening for blood, sugar, bacteria.
- Ultrasound.
- Check for fetal heartbeats.
- Assessment of uterine size.

What You and Your Doctor May Discuss

What Your Doctor Can Offer

As we saw in Chapter 5, different doctors offer different levels of technology and expertise when it comes to multiple pregnancies. When your twins, triplets, or quads are diagnosed, you may want to reconsider your practitioner and where you want to deliver, or at least assure yourself that the arrangements you have made are appropriate to your new condition. Women who have been treated by a fertility specialist—usually a reproductive endocrinologist—will want to find out their doctor's plans for the transition to an ob/gyn, which may occur as soon as the pregnancy is confirmed or which might take place as late as 10 to 12 weeks, when the viability of the pregnancy is assured.

The Doctor–Patient Relationship

Eventually, you'll choose the doctor you want to take you to delivery—and both of you will need to know what the ground rules are. This is when you'll want to ask the kinds of questions we discussed in Chapter 5—when you should call, what to do in case of emergency, what philosophy and values each of you holds, what you expect from each other. If you do want to change doctors, it's obviously better to do so as soon as possible; on the other hand, if you're going to stay with your current doctor, it's good to know what he or she expects from you. This is also the time when your doctor will review with you what you can expect over the next ten months—the schedule of office visits, the changes in your body, the various plans for delivery, the kinds of support available after the baby is born. I suggest talking about this visit ahead of time with your partner and with any trusted friends who've given birth, so that you come in calm, relaxed, and with a written list of questions. That way, you and your doctor can use this time as efficiently as possible, and you can leave the doctor's office happy and assured of good prenatal care.

Your Type of Twinning

As we saw in Chapter 2, the type of twinning—mono- or diamnionic, mono- or dichorionic—is very important in determining possible problems in the pregnancy and delivery. The optimum time to determine chorionicity is probably at 10 to 11 weeks, where there is high precision and the test is quick and easy. Your doctor needs to know what type of twins you've got to determine what he or she should watch out for as the pregnancy progresses. For more on what your doctor—and you—will want to know, see Chapter 2.

Your Family History

In Chapters 2 and 6, we talked about the various types of genetic conditions that might be passed on, as well as the various responses you and your partner might choose. The process of knowing what your situation is and deciding what to do about it will likely continue throughout your first trimester, but you can begin by sharing with your doctor all the information you have about your and your partner's genetic histories.

Screening for Abnormalities

There is a wide range of ways to screen for possible problems with one or more of your multiples, depending on your age, your partner's age, and your family histories:

- **Maternal serum screening or "triple screen."** This test of the mother's blood can be done as early as 15 weeks to screen for structural abnormalities. For more about this test, see Chapter 6.
- **Chorionic villus sampling (CVS).** CVS is done most safely at Week 10 or 11. If you have a high risk of carrying a fetus with a genetic disease, I would recommend this procedure. CVS screens

for genetic problems in the fetus, including both chromosomal disorders (for example, Down's syndrome) and single-gene defects (sickle-cell anemia, Tay-Sachs, Canavan, and the like). The test involves a catheter inserted through the cervix—or a needle into the abdominal wall—and into the placenta between the uterus and the chorion, depending on the location of the placenta. The point of this procedure is to sample the *villi*—fetal blood vessels that extend into the placenta and are bathed with the mother's blood. In multiple pregnancies, a sample must be taken for each fetus, though about 1 percent of the time it's not possible to get tissue from more than one fetus. Results of the test are usually available within a week. This is typically a very reliable test, though there may be a risk of one twin's sample contaminating the other's; however, this is less common with today's more careful sonographic mapping of the location of each fetus. The risk of miscarriage is about 1 percent as opposed to a risk of 0.5 to 1 percent for amniocentesis—which may not be significantly different. However, you can't have amnio until close to Week 15, so if you're considering a reduction or abortion, you may want this information earlier. It's still being debated whether CVS poses an increased risk for twins or other multiples. For more on CVS and how it can enhance your choices, see Chapter 6.

- **First-trimester sonogram for chromosomal abnormalities.** One of the most exciting recent advances in diagnostic procedures is the discovery that the size of the back of your babies' necks gives us important information about their condition. It seems that a thickness of three millimeters or more during the first trimester is associated with a higher rate of chromosomal abnormalities. Your doctor may use the noninvasive fetal nuchal translucency measurement—measuring the thickness of your babies' necks and looking for fluid—to glean additional information about their condition.

- **Amniocentesis.** This test isn't safe until Week 15, and most women have it sometime between their 15th and 18th weeks. For more on amniocentesis, see the next chapter.

Urinary-Tract Infections

Even if you don't have symptoms, you might have an *asymptomatic* urinary-tract infection (UTI), which, as we saw earlier, puts you at increased risk of a kidney infection. Infections in the vagina, urethra, or bladder also create an increased risk of preterm labor, so it's important to test for such infections and catch them in the early stages. That's why your monthly office visit always includes a urine sample. (For more on infections and preterm labor, see Chapter 14.)

If you do have a UTI, your doctor may prescribe *ampicillin,* a pregnancy-safe derivative of penicillin, or *Macrodantin,* a nonpenicillin antibiotic used for those who are allergic to penicillin. *Cephalosporin* and other so-called "broader spectrum" antibiotics (that is, antibiotics used for a wide range of purposes) can also be used during pregnancy. *Ciprofloxacin* and all floxacin derivatives are not at all safe during pregnancy, even though they are routinely used to treat UTIs in nonpregnant adults.

If you do have a UTI, be sure to take all the medication your doctor prescribes. It's tempting to stop when the symptoms disappear—but don't give in to temptation! The infection can persist without symptoms, putting you at exactly the same risk as before.

Even while taking medication, treat your UTI by drinking plenty of water, which helps to flush the bacteria out of your system. Cranberry juice is also helpful, because it alters the pH (acidity) of your urine, making it a less hospitable environment for bacteria. If you get frequent UTIs during your pregnancy, you may be given preventive antibiotics.

Miscarriage

If you've had a history of miscarriage, or if you've got any uterine abnormalities—a double uterus, a heart-shaped uterus, or uterine septum (divider)—your doctor may want you to be on the lookout for the following symptoms of miscarriage:

• **Bleeding.** Although some bleeding may occur during the first few months of pregnancy, you should keep your doctor in-

Cutting-Edge Science:
New Diagnostic Tests Are on the Way

One of the most exciting new developments in prenatal care is the *fetal nuchal translucency measurement,* a test that uses sonography to measure the thickness of a special area behind the baby's neck. In England, where this technique was developed and where it is taught in a highly standardized way, this measurement has proven to be a remarkably effective means of predicting chromosomal problems, picking up some 80 percent of all Down's syndrome cases. The test needs to be validated in the United States, though, before becoming standard practice.

Another type of diagnosis involves screening the mother's blood for molecules of fetal blood that have entered the mother's circulation. If these fetal blood cells can be screened for chromosomal abnormalities, this test can replace amniocentesis and other types of early screening—and greatly increase the pickup rate for chromosomal problems. Again, this is still all experimental.

Finally, tests that check for PAPP-A, a substance that the placenta produces, and hCG, a hormone in the mother's blood, might also help with first-trimester Down's syndrome screening and are under investigation.

formed, especially if the bleeding continues for more than a few days. If you're bleeding as heavily as you do during your period—that is, if you need to use a menstrual pad—call your doctor right away. However, remember that up to one-third of all women pregnant with multiples have some bleeding during the first trimester, and most of them end up having perfectly normal pregnancies. Just call your doctor, who will do an ultrasound to rule out any problems.

If you pass grayish or pink tissue, or blood clots, you may already have begun to miscarry. Try to save any material that passes out of your body, as it may help your doctor understand both what has happened and what your current situation is. And, of course, call your

First-Trimester Bleeding: What Does It Indicate?

- **Bright-red blood**—active bleeding.
- **Dark staining**—blood that is making its way out from the cervix and vagina. Sometimes blood known as *subchorionic* or *retroplacental collection* gathers behind the placenta and takes several weeks to be reabsorbed. Meanwhile, some of the blood may pass out through the cervix and vagina.
- **Cramping and pain.** Either mild or severe cramping might indicate a miscarriage.
- **Fever.** Not all fevers indicate a miscarriage, of course, but let your doctor know what's going on, especially if you have any of the other symptoms on this list.

doctor. If you can't reach him or her right away, consider that you're experiencing a medical emergency and follow the procedure you've agreed upon.

If your doctor does want you to come to the office or go to a hospital, you can expect the following procedure:

- Someone will take your vital signs, including pulse and blood pressure.
- You'll get a pelvic exam to see if there is any tissue or blood clots.
- Your uterus and abdomen will be examined.
- Your doctor will evaluate your cervix to see whether it is open (evidence of a miscarriage) or closed.
- You will probably have a transvaginal ultrasound.

Depending on what your doctor finds, he or she may suggest one of several courses:

- Further tests to confirm rising hormone levels (evidence of continuing pregnancy).
- Decreased activity and/or bed rest until the bleeding stops.

- Progesterone supplements to prevent miscarriage—a controversial procedure, since many doctors don't believe this is an effective treatment.

Even if you've had some bleeding, there are grounds for great optimism if the bleeding is *acute and finite*—that is, if it does not continue throughout your pregnancy. And if your embryos or fetuses are the right size for your length of pregnancy, you're entitled to feel even more confident.

My patient Dolores was 37 when she got pregnant with twins due to a combination of Pergonal and a technique known as *intravenous insemination*. She and her husband had been trying to conceive for some five years before they turned to fertility treatments, and although I wasn't her doctor during that time, I wondered if the problems she'd had conceiving might also lead to problems carrying to term. I didn't want to alarm her, but I did want her to be well-versed in the possible signs of miscarriage.

Dolores was spotting throughout her first month—another reason I wanted to keep a close eye on her. When she called me during her second month with severe cramping, I told her to come in right away. Her husband came with her into the examining room, and I could see that all three of us feared the worst.

In fact, the situation was serious—Dolores had a small blood clot behind the placenta (subchorionic or retroplacental collection)—but the ultrasound revealed that both of her babies were doing fine. I prescribed bed rest just to be on the safe side, and she was happy to comply. Two weeks later, sonograms revealed that the blood clot had shrunk considerably, and Dolores was able to get out of bed and engage in nonstrenuous activity. By her third month, the blood clot was gone, the babies were well, and Dolores was even able to return to her job as a data systems analyst, after promising me that she'd take frequent breaks throughout the day and put her feet up during an extra-long lunch hour. (Luckily, her boss and colleagues were happy to cooperate.) Dolores delivered on the early side—at 32 weeks—but her twin boy and girl were healthy and beautiful.

Brooke wasn't so lucky. Her first pregnancy—conceived at age

28—ended in a miscarriage during her third month. I couldn't find any reason for the unhappy event, so I concluded that this was one of the many unexplained miscarriages that probably indicate some kind of structural or chromosomal problem with the fetus.

Brooke understood intellectually that her miscarriage might have been nature's way of taking care of a fetus that simply wasn't equipped to survive—but emotionally she mourned the loss of her pregnancy. She successfully gave birth to twins the following year, and she continues to be delighted with her daughters, who are now four years old and doing fine. Still, she told me, every year when the anniversary of her miscarriage comes around, she finds herself feeling a little sad, wondering about the child she lost.

Loss of One Fetus

Sometimes a pregnancy is only partially lost. And sometimes the ultrasound diagnosis only *seems* to show two or more babies. One study found that 21.8 percent of twin pregnancies diagnosed in the first trimester went on to deliver only one twin.

The National Collaborative Perinatal Project reports that some 33 singletons are lost per 1,000 births, whereas the comparable loss rate for twins—once the pregnancy is well-established—is 139 per 1,000, with a rate 2.7 times higher for monozygotic than for dizygotic twins. (For more on zygosity, see Chapter 3.) However, most of these higher mortality rates were related not to the early loss of a twin, but to the death of low-birth-weight infants, primarily because twins tend to be delivered earlier and at lower birth weights than their singleton counterparts.

If you do experience the symptoms of a miscarriage, you may still be carrying one or more multiples. Sometimes, too, the loss of a multiple shows up only on the ultrasound—another reason why your doctor will probably be giving you regular monthly sonograms.

The loss of a fetus or an embryo is never easy, even if one or more unborn children remain. However, when this loss occurs during the first trimester, it is more than likely to be related to a genetic or chromosomal defect, a structural problem, or a problem of the placenta—all of which would probably cause trouble later in the pregnancy, during birth, or in the child's life.

While this may be difficult to accept, its corollary is somewhat more comforting: The babies who do survive after an early loss have a high chance of continuing the pregnancy without complications and of being born as healthy, thriving children. The loss of one or more multiples later on in gestation does put the surviving fetus(es) at higher risk of preterm labor. But, as we'll see in Chapter 15, we're often able to manage preterm labor and still achieve good outcomes for both mother and babies.

Jennifer was a single mother who had used ART to help her conceive and found herself pregnant with triplets. At age 29, she was highly committed to having a child, and after the initial shock of her multiple pregnancy had worn off, she started getting ready to welcome *three* children. She experienced severe cramping in her third month, however, and when we rushed her to the hospital, the ultrasound revealed that her triplet pregnancy had been spontaneously reduced to twins.

"Logically, I know it was for the best," Jennifer told me when I saw her recently. "My two boys are a real handful, and I don't know how I would have managed with three, especially if the third one had had special problems—or whatever ended up causing the loss.

"Still, it *was* a loss. I don't think about it all that often, but sometimes I find myself wondering what the third baby would have been like. And I wonder if somehow Jonny and Jason miss their brother, if somehow they realize that they lost him, even at such an early age."

Coping with a Loss

If you suffer from the loss of one or more of the fetuses you are carrying, you might need to find ways to mourn and cope with the loss. While some women experience no emotional aftereffects from a miscarriage, others find the loss all the more difficult because it is often unrecognized: Partners may not realize how traumatic the change can be, particularly if one or more fetuses still survive, while friends and family may not even have known about the pregnancy.

Some women find they need a special ritual—a kind of funeral ceremony—to help them honor and let go of the potential child they were carrying. Other women simply need time to process the experience, by spending time alone in a favorite place, writing in their journal, or talking things over with their partner or friends. Still other women benefit from counseling, both because of the specific advice of the counselor and because the very act of going for help is a way of acknowledging the seriousness of what has happened, especially if the loss has been kept private. Whatever your style of mourning may be, make time to process your loss so that you can move on to enjoy the children who remain or who will come in the future.

How Your Babies Are Developing

If your doctor showed you your ultrasound at four weeks, what you'd see is either one or two little sacs (depending on if your babies are monochorionic or dichorionic; see Chapter 3). Your twins are already swimming in their amniotic sacs of fluid, but during the fourth week these aren't visible yet.

From Week 4 through Week 8, your twins begin to develop brains, bladders, kidneys, livers, reproductive tracts, spines, hearts, arms, and legs, pretty much at the same rate as singletons. By Week 6½, the ultrasound will show you a tiny embryo or two, about two or three millimeters long—smaller than a grain of rice. You can not only see the fetuses, you can check the fetal yolk sacs and hearts. By Week 7 or 8, each twin is the size of *two* grains of rice, and their heartbeats show up on the ultrasound.

As your multiples reach the end of your first trimester, they cease to be embryos and start becoming fetuses. Their kidneys, intestines, arms, and legs are still developing. And they more than double their size between Week 8 and Week 12—from four to nine centimeters. Their weight gain is even more dramatic, from one gram at Week 8 to 20 grams by Week 12. By Week 12 you can hear the fetuses' heartbeats by Doptone.

11.

What's Happening to Your Body?: The Second Trimester

❧

I *loved* my second trimester!" Marsha exults. "All right, yes, I was big as a house, and my colleagues kept giving me funny looks whenever they thought I didn't notice. But I had so much *energy*! I loved my job, I loved my body, and I had these two wonderful babies to look forward to. For those three months, I was sitting on top of the world."

"That second trimester was definitely the best of the three," admits Miriam. "I hated feeling fat, and Ira and I were constantly fighting about money—I think it had finally hit us that we were going to have two children to support. But I must confess, there was a big part of me that really got into all the fixing and planning—getting the nursery ready, baby-proofing the house, buying little baby clothes. You'd told me not to leave any of that too long, and I was *so* glad I took your advice, because by my third trimester I was doing all those last-minute things at work, plus I had a lot less energy."

"Finally, I could eat again!" recalls Sarah. "My morning sickness *did* last into my fourth month, but things were so much better by Month Five! And Philip and I were finally starting to believe that we really *would* have three children. We were still scared, but also so relieved."

Most women find that the second trimester is the honeymoon time in pregnancy. The nausea and vomiting (usually) diminish; hormonal changes tend to elevate your mood; you've settled into the news; and you've got more information on your babies' condition. You'll probably feel more energized, though as a multiple mom, you'll still need plenty of rest.

This is a good time for planning and preparation: arranging your household, talking with your other children, getting ready for your absence at work, and joining with your partner to put together the support system you'll both need as your pregnancy progresses. This is also the time to make final preparations for your birth and delivery, if you haven't already done so. You don't know what kinds of rest and quiet your doctor may be prescribing in your third trimester as the two of you work to extend your term to its optimal time. And of course, despite all your best efforts, your twins very well might come early. So whatever needs to be done, do it now!

Although as a multiple mom, you'll probably have been gaining weight—noticeably, by this time—the second trimester is when the pregnancy really begins to show. Some women find this extremely gratifying: For the first time in their lives, instead of feeling "fat," they can feel pregnant. Other women find their new body image upsetting. Perhaps it confirms that they really *are* pregnant, bringing up fears and anxieties that had been buried until now. Perhaps it makes them feel far too much like their own mothers, a shift in identity that they weren't prepared for. Or perhaps, after a lifetime of dieting and concern about their weight, they do indeed feel "fat," and they resent the "bloated, heavy" way they look and feel.

Certainly a woman can have any or all of these feelings and still be overjoyed about the upcoming birth. And most assuredly, the pregnancy-related mood swings and fatigue that you may be feeling throughout your pregnancy (though probably less so in this trimester) only add to the emotional roller coaster. (I found it telling that when Annie, perfect mom and minister's wife on the TV show *Seventh Heaven,* got pregnant with her twins, she became all but impossible to live with.)

As always, try to keep a sense of perspective—and a sense of humor. And do keep the lines of communication open: with your doctor, your partner, your family, and your friends. If ever there was a time to draw on the support systems in your life, this is it!

"Sometimes I felt like we had turned into something out of *Little House on the Prairie,*" Zoe confesses. "We had our weekly family meetings—once he got the idea, Sean absolutely insisted on meeting every Sunday night, and sometimes he'd call a meeting during the week too. I had asked the kids' favorite aunt, Rosie, to do something with either Sean or Lissa once a weekend, so they wouldn't feel neglected. And Nick and I were going to a twins' support group. Both our parents live in other cities, but you better believe they each found time to come and visit—though I can't complain, because Nick's parents left us a freezer full of food, and mine took me shopping for baby furniture. The support was great—but sometimes I missed the days when I just got to go for a walk or spend some time by myself."

What You May Notice

- **Renewed appetite.** Usually, by the second trimester, the vomiting and nausea are over, and your appetite returns. In fact, you may feel like eating everything in sight! Don't worry—your babies need lots of food, and the only way they can get it is for you to eat. Follow your appetite, and your cravings. If your cravings feel extreme or long-lasting, you should tell your doctor, so that he or she can prescribe vitamin or mineral supplements if necessary.
- **Less-frequent urination.** You'll be urinating more often than before you were pregnant, but probably not as often as during your first trimester. You'll probably still have to get up a few times during the night, but you'll be on a much more normal schedule during the day. ("Thank heavens!" Rosario says about this particular feature of the second trimester. "My clients were *very* patient with me, even if most of them didn't know *why* I was suddenly interrupting our sessions to run to the bathroom. But was I relieved to be able to make it through a forty-five-minute counseling session!")
- **Constipation.** This problem, which may have begun during the first trimester, is likely to get worse now. Drink lots of water, eat

plenty of fiber, and, if necessary, ask your doctor about a fiber supplement. Ideally, you'll be moving your bowels at least once a day.

- **Sleep changes.** Some women notice more dreaming and/or more vivid dreams. "I started keeping a dream journal, which I still keep," Natalie told me. "I felt like all of a sudden I had this wonderful secret life." Jeannette, on the other hand, says, "I've never been very good without my eight hours, and now it seemed like I was tossing and turning all night long." Restlessness is also a usual part of this stage of pregnancy, as you continue to seek new positions that will be comfortable for your ever-changing body.
- **Vaginal discharge.** Higher estrogen levels during the second trimester may cause you to produce a white, creamy vaginal discharge.
- ➤ ALERT: If you have burning or itching associated with vaginal discharge, it may be vaginitis and require treatment. If you have a big gush of fluid or blood, tell your doctor right away.
- **A change in headache patterns.** Some women report more headaches during pregnancy; others notice that they have headaches less frequently. If you're one of those who has more headaches than usual during pregnancy, you'll probably notice the increase during the second trimester. Drink plenty of fluids—and start to notice what physical or emotional triggers can set off a headache. Some women have particular trouble with migraine headaches. For more on coping with migraines during pregnancy, see Chapter 8.
- ➤ ALERT: No matter what your headache patterns were before pregnancy, if you notice an increase in the frequency and/or severity of headache pain, tell your doctor. And, of course, don't take *any* medication—except Tylenol—without your doctor's approval.
- **Dramatically expanded abdomen.** Every pregnant woman starts showing eventually, of course, but multiple moms "expand" earlier, and more. Practically speaking, you'll be going through more size changes than singleton moms, so *do* splurge on some nice maternity clothes, but also be creative. Borrow your hus-

band's clothes (some people think it's sexy!), ask different-sized friends for their old maternity wear, bargain-hunt for the local maternity shop with the most reasonable prices. "I really got caught by surprise," Zoe admits. "I hadn't changed size all *that* much with Lissa and Sean, but the twins were a whole different ball game. I remember looking in my closet and realizing that the clothes I thought were going to get me all the way through the pregnancy were just about enough for the first six months. Luckily, there was still some money in our pregnancy budget." (See Figure 1.)

- **Noticeably enlarged breasts.** Make sure your bras are giving you adequate support, with straps that go around the shoulders and back. You'll probably need to buy special maternity bras; to economize, see if you can find the kind that double as nursing bras.

- **Swelling feet.** *Increased peripheral edema*—that is, increased swelling in the peripheral areas of your body—includes swelling feet, which can change whole shoe sizes between morning and evening. Make comfortable shoes—not fashion—your priority until after delivery! And put your feet up—that is, higher than your heart—as often as possible, but for at least a couple of hours each day. "You really stressed that, Dr. Leiter," Jeannette recalls, "and I'm so glad. Because you were so tough with me, I had the courage to be a bit more assertive at work than I normally would have been. I hated the thought that my boss might come into my office and find me with my feet up on my desk. But I just kept telling myself, 'My doctor says I have to—it's a medical necessity.' "

- **Increased curve of the spine.** Because of the increased weight in your abdomen, your spine tends to curve more than it otherwise would, a condition known as *lordosis*. It's better for the long-term health of your back—as well as for your short-term comfort—if you stay away from high heels.

- **Mood changes.** As we saw in Chapter 10, both PMS and pregnancy are marked by hormonal swings that can create extreme, sudden, or frequent mood changes—not to mention the fact that your life is about to change! See Chapter 4 for some ways to nurture yourself and to ask for support from your partner, family,

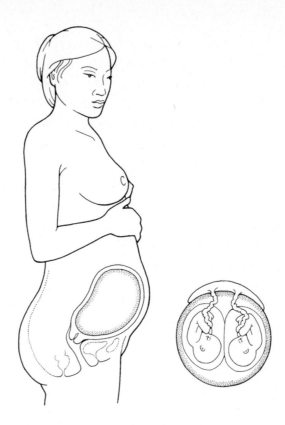

FIGURE 1. The Second Trimester

and friends. Plenty of rest, de-stressing exercises, meditation, and moral support can help you—and your loved ones—ride out the mood changes.

- **Fetal movement.** As you move into the last month of this trimester, you should notice your twins moving every day. If you feel movement on one side only, don't worry—both sets of legs may be facing the same way! As with singletons, quickening in a multiple pregnancy takes place sometime between 17 and 21 weeks. You may be feeling *more* movement than with a singleton pregnancy, but you won't be feeling it any earlier.
- **Edema, or swelling.** As the pregnancy progresses, fluid may collect in your connective tissues, causing various parts of your body to swell. Some women get *carpal tunnel syndrome:* a numb

or tingling feeling in the palm and fingers caused by the compression of nerves within the wrist. This syndrome almost always disappears by two weeks after delivery. If you are experiencing edema of any kind, including swollen feet, your doctor will probably recommend rest, putting your feet up (higher than your heart) for a couple of hours each day—and no restriction of fluids. The swelling indicates that your tissues are collecting water, rather than using it efficiently. If you have carpal tunnel syndrome, you can buy wrist splints at the pharmacy to relieve some of the pressure. Try to sleep with your hands higher than your heart.

- **Overheating.** Also toward the end of the trimester, you are probably starting to feel hotter than usual, since your metabolic rate while at rest is speeding up. This warm sensation is nothing to worry about, but do make sure to drink enough water to replace any fluids you lose by sweating.

- **Cramps in the calf.** Being awakened from a sound sleep by leg cramps is a condition not confined to pregnancy, but for some reason, pregnant moms are at special risk. One theory is that cramping is caused by a shortage in calcium or potassium, so make sure your diet is well balanced. And of course, talk to your doctor. For the cramp itself, straighten your leg and flex your ankle, so that your foot is perpendicular to your leg. You or your partner can also gently stroke the long muscle in your calf. Some women need to walk off the cramp for an hour or two the next morning.

- **Varicose veins.** Women carrying multiples tend to get varicose veins earlier than in other pregnancies, as the increased blood volume in your body may cause your blood vessels to swell. Support hose and resting for a few hours a day with your feet elevated will help stabilize your blood flow.

➢ ALERT: If your veins or legs seem unusually swollen, or if you notice heat, redness, or tenderness in your legs or elsewhere, tell your doctor immediately. You may have phlebitis (superficial or deep inflammation of the veins).

You may also have ongoing symptoms from the first trimester:

- Increased appetite.
- Fatigue.
- Heartburn and indigestion.
- Constipation.
- Dry mouth.
- Extra saliva.
- Stuffiness.
- Nosebleeds.
- Swollen and/or bleeding gums.
- Hemorrhoids.
- Breathlessness.
- Elevated heart rate.
- Breast tenderness and changes in appearance.
- Swollen feet.
- Changes in sexual feelings.
- Sensitive skin.
- Stretch marks.
- Anemia.

Tips for Coping

- By the fourth or fifth month, multiple moms tend to be so big that many people assume they're at least six or seven months along. Some women get tired of correcting well-meaning strangers who make this assumption—so they just let the mistake stand.
- You'll probably need two to three different sets of maternity clothes (one of my patients called them "large," "extra large," and "enormous"!), since your shape will change more than the mother of a singleton. If your friends are giving you their hand-me-downs, see if you can get contributions from different-size friends. Shopping for maternity clothes by catalog can save you time as well as wear and tear on your feet. See the Resources section for some shop-by-mail (or Internet) suggestions.

- Birth classes can be an invaluable help in preparing for a multiple delivery, even if you've already given birth. If you're carrying multiples, you want to start those classes early: Whereas singleton parents are targeted for delivery at 40 weeks, your target date is closer to 36 weeks (earlier if you're carrying triplets or quads), and you also face greater risk of premature delivery. Parents who have already given birth may find that they still have more to learn, while both first-timers and veterans will appreciate the informal support group that knowing other pregnant couples provides. Some areas feature special birth classes geared to parents of multiples, which offer even more specific support. Most birth classes help to educate the family, teach the woman relaxation techniques, and create a close, trusting relationship between the mother and her birth coach. By the way, if you're on bed rest, you may be able to find instructors who come directly to your home. And many hospitals offer videos on labor, childbirth, and newborn care.

- How do you cope with the cosmetic and health problems of varicose veins? I'm sorry to report that one crucial way involves support hose. Okay, so they're nobody's idea of a fashion statement and they're hot and uncomfortable in the summer, but you've only got two legs, and support hose are the way to take care of them. You might begin your pregnancy with the hose you find at your local maternity store or surgical-supply outlet, but your belly will eventually be quite large in relation to your legs, so toward the third trimester you may need to get your hose custom-made. Ask your doctor to recommend a vendor. By your second trimester, you need to put these stockings on first thing in the morning, before your feet hit the floor. In fact, you should lie in bed for another 15 minutes or so before you stand up. By the way, during *my* pregnancies, I wore surgical scrubs whenever I could—that way, the support hose didn't show!

What Your Doctor's Visits Will Include

In your sixth month, your doctor may begin to schedule your visits every two weeks instead of every three to four weeks.

Your Childbirth-Class Catalog

There are several types of childbirth preparation currently being taught. Here are three of the best-known:

- **Lamaze**—This technique is based on the principle that shallow, rapid breathing will help you through the pain. You learn how to concentrate and relax by rehearsing certain responses to contractions, on the theory that, like an athlete, your planned responses will override the impulse to give in to the pain. You work closely with a coach who helps you first practice, then apply, the techniques.
- **Bradley**—In this method, you learn deep abdominal breathing and relaxation, as expressed in the phrase "Breathe into the pain." Rather than ignoring your bodily sensations by concentrating on breathing—as in Lamaze—you use your breath to focus on what actually *is* happening in your body. Your partner is there to help you focus. Some Bradley method teachers are emphatic about making it through a labor with no medication, but for many mothers—especially multiple moms—this isn't an option. Either way, the techniques can be helpful.
- **Grantly Dick-Read**—This method is based on the premise that labor pains come from the mother's fear of the unknown. The goal of these childbirth classes, then, is to educate the mother—and perhaps also her partner—about what she can expect, helping her to enter labor in a more relaxed state.

- **Pelvic exam.** In your fourth month, your doctor will want to make sure that your uterus is growing as it should. Given that twins have a higher rate of preterm labor and passive cervical dilation (that is, cervical dilation *not* marked by pain or discharge), your doctor will also want to be sure that your cervix is the right length and size for your gestational date and to check how dilated you are by pelvic exam. A transvaginal sonogram may be used to check your cervix's length as well.
- **Glucose screening.** Sometime between Weeks 24 and 28, your doctor will probably do a glucose screening to make sure you aren't experiencing gestational diabetes. If you have a family his-

tory of diabetes or are having particular symptoms, he or she may do this test even earlier.

- **Blood test for hemoglobin.** If your doctor is concerned about anemia, he or she may test your hemoglobin (red blood cell) levels.
- **Tests in response to particular symptoms, especially swelling or edema.**
- **Assessment of weight gain.**
- **Blood-pressure test.**
- **Evaluation of pulse and respiratory rate.**
- **Fundal height of the uterus.**
- **Physical assessment of your breasts.**
- **Urine sample—screening for blood, sugar, bacteria.**
- **Ultrasound.**
- **Check for fetal heartbeats.**

What You and Your Doctor May Discuss

Weight Gain

As we saw in Chapter 7, early, adequate weight gain is crucial to the health of your multiples—and this is the trimester when the weight gain will really take off. If you're not gaining enough weight, your doctor may be concerned.

Although Shana and I had discussed at length the reasons her twins needed lots of nourishment early in the pregnancy, it was still hard for her to overcome the habits of a lifetime and commit to gaining the weight that her babies needed. "It's not just ego, it's my job," she would say whenever the topic of gaining weight came up. "If I'm ever going to get back to work once the babies are born, I can't afford to put on too much weight now."

Finally, I found some pictures of underweight premature twins and triplets and showed them to Shana, along with some photographs of multiples who had also been born early but who had good weights for their ages. "This is what we're up against," I told her. "It's not a question of your ego *or* your job. It's a question of what your babies will weigh if they're born early."

As soon as Shana saw what was at stake, her eating habits changed. She began making a positive effort to gain weight along the schedule that we'd worked out. As it happened, her babies *were* born on the early side—at 30 weeks—but at the respectable weights of 4 and 4½ pounds. Both of us were enormously relieved that she'd given them the wherewithal to survive and thrive despite their premature arrival.

Exercise

Although you need to be careful about what kinds of demands you place on your body, most doctors will encourage you to pay special attention to your exercise plan at this point in your pregnancy. Not only will moderate exercise help you get your figure back after the babies are born, but attention to the abdominal muscles now will pay off when you're in labor.

Rosario had never been fond of exercise, but she brought the same dogged determination to her pregnancy exercise plan that she'd shown when she came in for preconceptional counseling with a list of questions in her hand. She found time to swim for 20 minutes each day and religiously followed a routine of stretches and back exercises. I was glad she was taking steps to make her pregnancy, delivery, and postpartum recovery smoother and more comfortable.

Your Travel Schedule

I personally don't advise long-distance air travel after the 20th week of a multiple pregnancy, for several reasons: It's stressful, you're going far away from your doctor, and you might have to carry heavy luggage. If you must travel, make sure you and your doctor agree on how much and under what circumstances.

Business travel was a big issue for Marsha, of course, as she frequently flew halfway around the world to supervise her three overseas factories. Typically, she found many creative ways to minimize the strains: She arranged for her assistant to ship ahead most of what she needed, so she didn't have to deal with luggage, and she brought re-

---

Watch Your Diet!

Your second trimester is a good time to review your diet. Remember, your weight gain is directly correlated to your babies' weight gain, so you should make sure that you're getting adequate nutrition and enough calories to support your multiple pregnancy.

Remember to get enough protein and calcium, as well as taking your vitamins, folic acid, and iron if necessary.

If you've got any questions about what you should be eating, check with your ob/gyn. If you're having trouble figuring out your diet, a nutritionist can help.

---

laxation tapes to help her sleep on the plane and in strange hotel rooms.

Still, the strain of travel, the demands of a twin pregnancy, and Marsha's chronic hypertension were all cause for concern, and the day came when I had to strongly advise her against further travel during the remaining three and a half months of her pregnancy. I could see how much it cost this ambitious, powerful woman to relinquish the care of the company she had so carefully built, but she accepted the constraints calmly, if not always cheerfully. Remembering my own hectic schedule as a pregnant resident, I wondered if I would have been able to handle curtailing my professional activities as gracefully as she did. (For more about travel, see Chapter 9.)

How Much Rest You're Getting

As the second trimester progresses, you will probably find yourself needing more and more rest. Your doctor may make one or more of the following suggestions:

- cut back some of your usual activities;
- modify your work schedule;

- work from home part of the time;
- leave work early to beat the rush-hour commute;
- change responsibilities at work to allow for less time on your feet.

As you can see, I've had widely varying reactions from my patients when I encourage them to rest, from relief and gratitude to resentment and anxiety. Again, when I remember how lucky I was to be able to keep working, I empathize strongly with any patient who wants to keep up with her professional commitments. At the same time, it's my responsibility to remind my patients that a multiple pregnancy has special risks and demands—and that sometimes rest is called for. When I see the creativity and commitment that my patients bring to changing their work schedules, I am moved by the lengths to which women will go to ensure a safe and healthy pregnancy.

Your Babies' Condition

Your doctor will probably want to take an ultrasound sometime early in the second trimester, just to make sure that everything's okay. Your regular physical exam at that point will include a check for fetal heartbeats by Doptone, and your doctor may also want to check maternal serum alpha-fetoprotein (MSAFP) levels. (For more on this test, see Chapter 6.) As you approach Week 20, your doctor will want to give you an ultrasound to make sure that your babies are structurally sound and that each has access to enough amniotic fluid.

Your doctor will also be checking to make sure that your babies have good fine and gross motor tone. He or she will pay special attention to how they move and make breathing motions during ultrasound and how they respond to various stimuli.

Amniocentesis

For various reasons, you and your doctor may be considering the possibility of amniocentesis in the second trimester. Amnio is possible as early as Week 15, although most women who have it do so between Weeks 15 and 18.

Amnio is highly recommended for women over 32 or 33 carrying twins and women over 31 carrying triplets, as well as in situations when babies are fathered by a man over 50, or when either partner has a family history of genetic or chromosomal disorders. Amnio may also be used to confirm or further explore the results of a CVS, triple marker test, or fetal nuchal translucency measurement (the measurement of your babies' necks, which may indicate chromosomal abnormalities). (For more on those tests, see Chapter 6. For more on family histories, see Chapter 2.) Even if abortion or reduction is not an option for you, your doctor will benefit from knowing as much as possible about any chromosomal or structural abnormalities in your multiples, and you and your partner may appreciate the extra time to prepare for a child with special needs.

Amniocentesis involves inserting a thin, hollow needle through the abdomen and uterus into the amniotic sac of each multiple, in order to take a sample of the fluid. Typically, a little dye is inserted into the sac as well, so that the person doing the procedure can be sure that he or she has sampled fluid from each multiple's sac. (If your twins are monozygotic, it may be enough to take fluid from just one sac. For more on zygosity and what it means, see Chapter 3.) The person doing the procedure uses an ultrasound image for guidance in finding each fetus and placenta. Fetal cells found in the amniotic fluid can then be tested for chromosomal problems, with the results usually available in seven to ten days.

Amniocentesis carries a risk of miscarriage between 0.5 and 1 percent. The risks of miscarriage for multiples after amnio may be greater than in a singleton pregnancy—probably because the risk of miscarriage is generally greater than in a singleton pregnancy. Some women do feel mild cramps, like menstrual cramps, and in rare cases there may be slight leakage of amniotic fluid. Of course, you should tell your doctor about any symptoms you experience.

Miscarriage or the Loss of a Multiple

Although the possibilities of loss are drastically reduced during the second trimester, they do exist. Women whose twins are monochorionic are most vulnerable, with the rates of loss of a single twin ranging from 0.5 to 6.8 percent.

If a single twin is lost early in the pregnancy—say, by Week 12—the other's chances for survival are excellent, especially if the twins are dichorionic. (For more on chorionicity, see Chapter 3.) However, a twin lost after Week 20 significantly increases the risk to the other. In either case, though, there tends to be little risk to the health of the mother.

If you do lose a single fetus before Week 34, your doctor will be especially careful about monitoring the health and movement of the surviving fetus. As we've seen, you'll also want to attend to your emotional responses. If necessary, make sure you get the kind of counseling and support that you need to process the loss and to prepare yourself to welcome the child(ren) who do survive. (For more on miscarriage, loss, and mourning, see Chapter 10.)

Preterm Labor

Preventing preterm labor is probably your doctor's major concern at this point, since the longer your babies stay in the womb, the better their chances for health and survival. Sometime during your second trimester, your doctor will probably discuss with you the signs and symptoms of preterm labor: lower back pain, cramping, bloody discharge, leaking vaginal fluid, and repeated uterine tightening. This is another one of those "balancing acts" I've been talking about: You don't want to be panicking at every little twinge, but you *do* want to develop the greatest body awareness possible, since only you will be able to discern the first signs of preterm labor. For more on preventing and coping with preterm labor, see Chapter 14.

How Your Babies Are Developing

As your twins begin their second trimester, they're no longer embryos but fetuses, weighing an average of 20 grams apiece. As they begin Week 13, they're about one and a half inches long, resembling the "tadpole" shape of popular imagery. At this point, the babies' structural development is virtually done—now their growth involves getting larger and stronger. Although they can't yet move in any organized way, they do have reflexes, and ultrasound reveals that they move in the amniotic sac. In fact, when a needle is inserted for amniocentesis, we know that your twins will move away, and if you push on your abdomen during ultrasound, you can see them respond. You can also occasionally see them suck their thumbs! Your twins are making the transition to active beings who choose where, when, and how to move.

Over the first month of the trimester, each fetus will grow to weigh 120 grams—about four ounces—and measure about four inches. By Week 16, they can swallow, and their kidneys and their gastrointestinal systems are functioning. We can see water in their stomachs and urine in their bladders—urine that, when expelled, adds to the volume of amniotic fluid.

As your twins move on to Week 20, they grow from 16 to 25 centimeters—7½ inches. This is when you'll feel them move. Ultrasound will show you the thin, resilient membrane separating the two babies, who seem to be aware of each other as they frequently kick against the membrane. At this point, the babies cannot yet see or hear—but they do seem to yawn and then move their hands after yawning, in a way that is strikingly like the movement of newborns and infants.

By Week 20, each fetus is also producing most of its own amniotic fluid. Your babies are now structurally complete—except for the brain, which will continue to develop throughout the pregnancy.

Between Week 20 and Week 24, your babies will grow from about one pound to a pound and a half, some of which is a tiny bit of fat under the skin. At the end of the second trimester, they'll measure about a foot in length. By this point, your twins are in fairly constant contact as they kick each other through the resilient, elastic membrane that separates them. You may notice that they don't always have the same sleep schedules, so either one or both may be active.

During the last part of the second trimester, your twins will start to grow the soft, furry hair (*lanugo*) that you can see covering premature newborns. They'll also develop the *vernix caseosa,* a spongy substance produced by the cells of their skin to help keep them properly hydrated. By now, their joints flex and they're curled up in the classic fetal position. By the 24th week, your babies are approaching viability—if necessary, they might be able to survive outside of the womb. In fact, a significant proportion of 25-week fetuses do survive in today's NICUs (neonatal intensive-care units).

12

What's Happening to Your Body?:
The Third Trimester

⌒❦⌒

"Countdown time," Jeannette says ruefully when the subject of her third trimester comes up. "Suddenly it hit me that I was never going to *not* be a mother again. For the rest of my life, I'd have these children to take care of, to wonder about, to consider. I'd always been very close to my own mother, and I knew that parenting doesn't end when they turn eighteen—as far as I can see, it *never* ends."

"That third trimester is just a blur," Miriam recalls. "Ira and I were running around like a couple of chickens with our heads cut off, trying to get everything at work tied up before the kids showed up." I remember that I had to caution Miriam about taking it easier during her last trimester—as I'd so often had to remind other patients, who used *their* last three months to fix up their homes for the baby.

"Look," I've often told busy mothers-to-be, "your baby couldn't care less whether your baby's room is painted pink or blue, whether you've got decals up on the wall, or what kind of curtains you've got in there. Your baby could even sleep in a dresser drawer with a pad in it—so try to take advantage of your last few baby-free months."

"I *loved* being pregnant," Natalie says dreamily. "Even in that third trimester, when it was so hard to sleep and it seemed like I had to pee every five minutes. Yes, of course, I was looking forward to my babies, but in some other weird way, I think I just wanted to stay pregnant."

"Couldn't wait for it to be over," Rosario says briefly. "I was big, uncomfortable, having heartburn *all* the time. Honey, I was *over* it."

All mothers-to-be face a wide spectrum of conflicting emotions during their last three months of pregnancy. But multiple moms face a special challenge during this trimester: making it all the way through. Your twins are viable after about 24 weeks, but ideally they'll stay in the womb much longer than that. This is a time for taking excellent care of yourself, as you require both extra rest and extra help (carrying heavy objects and standing on your feet for long periods are both off-limits during these last three months!).

Like Jeannette and Miriam, Natalie and Rosario, most multiple moms I've known—myself included—have gone through a variety of feelings as the due date approaches: joy at the impending arrival of their twins, fears about managing multiple parenthood, a sense of disorientation and the inability to believe that one's life is going to change so radically. If you can possibly make some quiet time for yourself these days—time to write in a journal, have a heart-to-heart talk with a friend, or just "be" with yourself and your body—I strongly urge you to do so. Once your twins arrive, you'll be in the midst of a seemingly nonstop round of feedings and diaper changes, and the chance to ponder the meaning of this change will likely be out of reach for several months to come! So take time now. It's one of the best ways you can prepare yourself for the care of the new children who will soon be on their way.

What You May Notice

- **Increased weight.** For all pregnancies, and most especially for multiple ones, the third trimester is when the weight begins to affect the mother's back and legs, while the increased pressure from the uterus can also cause backaches. Your babies will be moving around a great deal, and their shifts in position will also affect how easily you're able to carry their additional weight. Warm baths are good for relieving backache and taking the strain off your abdomen, and by the time you're in your third trimester,

Questions for You and Your Partner to Consider

- Should we dress our twins alike or differently?
- Should we give them "related" names—Ben and Jen, Anna and Annette—or completely different names?
- Should we breast-feed or bottle-feed?
- Should they sleep together or in separate cribs?
- How will we handle that first month—hired help? Visiting relatives? Friends and neighbors? A doula? An au pair? If we'd like visitors but don't have the space for them, can we call on someone to help put people up? If we can't afford a full-time helper, can we find someone to come in for a few hours a day to cook and do some housework?
- Is this the time to find a twins' club or parents' support group?
- Can we spend some special time with our other children, to make up for the hectic time to come?
- If anyone is giving up his or her bedroom to make room for the twins, is this the time to move on that—rather than being surprised by a possible premature birth?
- What does our insurance cover? Will they pay "double" for two babies (two sets of shots, two sets of doctor visits, and so on)? If we've got two adults with two insurance policies, should we drop the second policy—or do the two policies together offer a better package?

you may be taking several baths a day. Don't indulge in the Jacuzzi, however, as its temperature is too hot for you and your babies. ("I just *lived* in the tub," Natalie recalls, while Jeannette, who was working full-time right up until her due date, says, "I made a beeline for the bathtub the minute I got home!") (See Figure 1.)

➤ ALERT: Tell your doctor about any new or unusual backache—it could be a sign of preterm labor. (For more on preterm labor, see Chapter 14.)

- **Pressure on the pelvis.** No mystery here—the babies are moving down into your pelvis, and of course you feel it!
- **Breathlessness.** Your uterus is so big, it's crowding your diaphragm, so you probably have more trouble than usual taking a

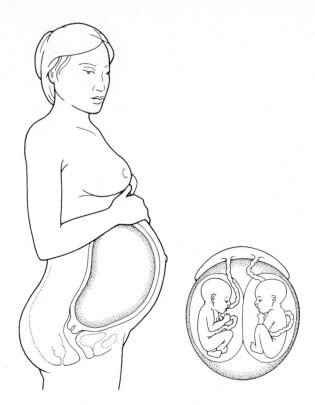

FIGURE 1. The Third Trimester

deep breath. Sitting upright rather than reclining may make it easier to breathe.

- **Frequent urination.** Although you got a respite in the second trimester, your bladder has even less room now. It fills up quickly, and you'll need to empty it frequently. ("At least now my clients knew *why* I was going to the bathroom so often!" Rosario says ruefully.)
- **Hemorrhoids.** You may notice more hemorrhoids as the trimester progresses. If you drink lots of water and eat lots of fiber, you'll address the constipation that might be a contributing factor. Your doctor may prescribe foam or suppositories. Cold packs—available without prescription from your drugstore; shaped like menstrual pads—can soothe the rectal area. Sitz baths (baths in Epsom salts and warm water)—two or three times a

day, for 15 to 20 minutes—can also bring relief. The baths are good for relieving backache too! ("With two children to take care of, even one bath a day seemed like an unimaginable luxury," Zoe recalls. "But Nick was great about making sure that I had at least fifteen minutes in the morning and fifteen minutes in the evening. The baths *did* help—but only while I was actually in them!")

- **Fatigue.** As you move through this trimester, you're likely to feel more and more tired. Be sure to give yourself frequent breaks, chances to put your feet up—and full permission to cancel out of family or social events!

- **Changes in the babies' movements.** In the second trimester, you may have noticed your babies' kicks and punches as they explored their new ability to move. As they move farther down into your pelvis, though, they're a bit more crowded, so the movement may seem more intense. By the middle of the third trimester, you probably notice certain predictable patterns in their movement. If you notice a new type of movement—repetitive and jerky—don't be concerned: One or both of your babies just has the hiccups!

- **Sleep discomfort.** Your vastly bigger body has a harder time finding a comfortable position in bed, although lots of pillows can help. Some women buy full-size body pillows that respond well to the body's various changes.

- **Braxton-Hicks contractions.** These contractions don't lead to labor—but they do involve the uterus, which may contract, as in a menstrual cramp, but without much pain. Multiple moms seem to get them more often than mothers who are carrying singletons. Sometimes you'll get one if you change your position—stand up, sit down, or lie down. Many women get them after orgasm, which is fine, as long as the contractions don't continue.

➤ ALERT: Up to three Braxton-Hicks contractions in an hour may be no problem, but if the contractions are painful, if you notice three or four in an hour—with or without pain—or if the contractions are accompanied by bleeding or leaking fluid, call your doctor right away. You might be experiencing preterm labor. (For more about preterm labor, see Chapter 14.)

- **Vaginal discharge.** You're probably noticing more white discharge than before your pregnancy. If you notice changes in discharge during this trimester—more abundant, accompanied by itching or burning or by changes in color—call your doctor. You might have a vaginal infection, which studies have shown can help set off preterm labor. It's fairly easy to treat bacterial infections in the vagina, however, so if you notice any changes, just let your doctor know. (For more on vaginal infections and preterm labor, see Chapter 14.)
- **Harder belly.** Up through the second trimester, your belly was getting bigger—but it was still soft and flexible. Now it's harder, like a soccer ball.

And, of course, you may continue to have ongoing symptoms from the second trimester:

- Increased appetite.
- Constipation.
- Heartburn and indigestion.
- Stuffiness.
- Nosebleeds.
- Swollen and/or bleeding gums.
- Elevated heart rate.
- Breast tenderness and changes in appearance; leakage from nipples.
- Changes in sexual feelings.
- Headaches.
- Sensitive skin.
- Stretch marks.
- Overheating.
- Anemia.
- Edema.
- Carpal tunnel syndrome.
- Leg cramps.
- Varicose veins.

Tips for Coping

- If you're having trouble with controlling your bladder, your doctor may recommend *Kegel* exercises. These exercises can be done anytime, anywhere, and will also help tone your uterine and vaginal muscles for delivery. You should clench the muscles around your vagina and anus, holding them tight for as long as possible, working your way up to about eight to ten seconds. Repeat at least 25 times at various times during the day.
- This isn't a bad time to start twin-proofing—you may not have the energy when the twins are actually home! Make sure there are no cords or wires near the twins' sleeping area, figure out what to do about pets, and check out your houseplants with the local nursery to find out which might be poisonous. I'd advise buying safety caps for all your electrical outlets, safety latches for your cabinets, and safety gates for your stairs and off-limits rooms. And, of course, start storing all poisons and toxic substances—including medications—in out-of-reach, locked cabinets.
- Buy two car seats now—*before* you're faced with the sudden problem of getting two babies home from the hospital! Federal regulations established in 1981 set the standards for car seats, so if you are making use of a hand-me-down, make sure it's no older than that. You might as well practice installing the car seats now too. If you've got two cars, make sure your car seats will fit in both—you never know what might happen in an emergency, and you must *never* do without a car seat or use an infant carrier in place of one. I recommend putting car seats in the backseat, always. For twins, put one seat in the center back and the other behind the right-hand passenger seat, so you can see both babies at all times. For babies under 20 pounds, the seats should go in backward. And, of course, never put a car seat in any seat that faces an airbag.
- Some parents prefer to put their twins in one crib; others go for separate sleeping arrangements. There are pros and cons to both arrangements: Together, they can more easily wake each other up, but they can also amuse each other before they wake *you* up. Either way, make sure the crib slats are no more than 2⅜ inches

apart (otherwise, a baby's head could get stuck) and that end posts are no higher than ⅟₁₆ inch above the crib's end panel (older children can strangle if their clothing gets caught on a post). Make sure, too, that the crib's mattress fits snugly and that the bumper pads—to protect the babies' heads—fit tightly around the crib. Cut the bumper ties as short as you can so your twins won't get tangled up in them.

- You're likely to get hours of use out of your stroller, so choose carefully. (If you already have a baby carriage, you can probably fit both newborns into it for a while—but you still might prefer buying a stroller before the babies arrive.) You'll find that you have a wide range of choices: twin strollers where the seats are side by side, two-seaters where the twins face each other, and even a three-seated stroller for your toddler to ride in as well. You'll also want a baby carrier—the front-facing sling that one baby can ride in, close to your body, so that your hands are free. I find it too hard to carry *two* babies that way, but you can buy twin front-packs if you like. Make sure that any carrier you buy is washable and has adjustable straps, and be sure it's durable—it's going to get plenty of wear! Find out when you buy it how the baby's head is supposed to be supported. And, of course, never use your carrier for anything other than walking with your baby—*never* for riding on a bike or in a car.
- This is the time to meet all the doctors who might be on call when you actually go into labor. Ask your own doctor who else might be delivering you, and find out how to meet with those physicians. You might go in with a list of preferences and strong concerns, so that you've had a chance to discuss these *before* you're all dealing with the actual delivery.

What Your Doctor's Visits Might Include

- **Pelvic exam**—In your seventh month, your doctor will want to find out whether your cervix is dilating.
- **Ultrasound**—Each month, your doctor will be making sure that each of your multiples has enough amniotic fluid and is growing well and at the same rate.

Stocking Up on Supplies

- **Bath supplies** might include two soft, hooded baby towels; several soft wash-cloths; and one bathtub or bath seat (you probably won't be washing the twins two at a time!).
- **Diapers** will go more quickly than you can imagine—ten a day per twin, at first. Whether you go with cloth diapers, disposables, or a diaper service, make sure you have a dozen extra cloth diapers on hand, just in case. They also make shoulder protectors for when you burp the babies. You might hint to coworkers, friends, or relatives that a year's worth of diaper service would make a great collective shower gift.
- **Clothing** is a tough call—the more clothes, the less washing, but also the more storage space and expense. At a minimum, each baby will need six cotton snap undershirts; six one-piece, leg-snap pajama sets; six receiving blankets; and two hats. If your babies are born in wintertime, they'll each need two blanket sleepers, two snowsuits, and two sets of booties (they may need those in summer too).

- **Blood test for hemoglobin**—Once again, to check for anemia, your doctor may test your hemoglobin (red blood cell) levels.
- **Nonstress test (NST)**—This is a common way for doctors to monitor fetal well-being. The idea is that the heart rate of a healthy fetus will accelerate with fetal movement. You might be asked to lie down in the doctor's office attached to a fetal monitor recording fetal heart rate and contractions and feel for fetal movements, pushing a button on a monitor each time you notice a movement. The tracing is checked for fetal heart rate accelerations that peak at 15 beats per minute above baseline and last 15 seconds. A reactive (or reassuring) test is one that has 2 or more such accelerations in 20 minutes. A nonreactive test is one without such accelerations over 40 minutes (which accounts for sleep-wake cycles). Sometimes one or two seconds of acoustic stimulation of the fetus/es may be done to wake up the babies and get a good reading.

- **Assessment of signs of preterm labor**—If you're showing any signs of preterm labor, or if you've had any history of preterm labor or premature birth in the past, your doctor will be monitoring you especially closely for signs of this condition. He or she may do a sonographic check of your cervical length, to make sure that your cervix is at least 30 millimeters long (a shorter cervix might indicate that your body is preparing to give birth). Another indicator of premature birth is your salivary estriol level—the level of estriols (a hormone) found in your saliva. If your estriols are at a normal level, you probably won't be delivering any time in the next two weeks, so depending on your likelihood of going into premature labor, your doctor may repeat this test every two weeks. A vaginal test can measure your levels of fetal fibronectin—another chemical whose levels can indicate imminent delivery. If your doctor is particularly concerned about premature labor, he or she may also recommend home uterine monitoring. (For more on this type of monitoring, and on premature labor in general, see Chapters 14 and 15.)
- **Assessment of weight gain.**
- **Blood-pressure test.**
- **Evaluation of pulse and respiratory rate.**
- **Physical assessment of your breasts.**
- **Urine sample**—**screening for blood, sugar, bacteria.**
- **Check for fetal heartbeats.**

What You and Your Doctor May Discuss

Your Energy Level

You're carrying around a lot more weight, and your body is still working hard to create two or more new lives. So if you're feeling fatigued and overwhelmed, relax—you're entitled! Your doctor will want to be sure that you're getting enough rest and that your job, household responsibilities, and exercise routine aren't putting undue strain on your already busy body.

"I thought I was going to keep working at least through my eighth month," Zoe recalls. "With Sean and Lissa, that's what I did.

But this time—no. It put a real strain on the family budget too, and at the worst possible time. But given how I was feeling, I really didn't have much choice."

"It's just a matter of being creative," Marsha insists, although she admits that her income level and the nature of her job allowed her a special freedom and flexibility that not many multiple moms enjoy. Still, when I hear her describe how she changed business meetings into teleconferences—"so I could make deals with my feet up, or even in bed!"—how she hired a new assistant to work with her at home, and how she had a masseuse come to her office each day for a special after-work pregnancy massage, I was impressed by her commitment to combine third-trimester rest periods with a full work schedule.

Your Babies' Weight

If your babies aren't gaining enough weight, your doctor may counsel you to eat more and rest more. This is a crucial time in building up your babies' birth weight, so work with your doctor to be sure that you're giving them all the support *they* need. (For more on nutrition and birth weight, see Chapter 7.)

By this point, Shana was fully committed to gaining the weight she needed—but I was still somewhat concerned. Since she seemed to be taking in the requisite number of calories, I asked her to add two rest periods to her schedule—two hours in the morning and another two in the evening. "I was so exhausted, I was happy to comply," Shana told me. "I wasn't working by then anyway, of course, and I think I had kind of pulled into myself by that point, gathering all my resources for the big event."

Your Babies' Condition

In singleton pregnancies, the doctor relies on the mother's ability to distinguish fetal movement. But in multiple pregnancies, the mother may not know which of her babies is moving, and her distended uterus makes it harder for her to be aware of fetal movement anyway. Your doctor may advise you to lie on your back and "listen" for movements from each fetus. Ideally, each fetus should move at least five times within 30 minutes. If you don't notice five movements per fetus, your doctor may want you to wait for a total of 60 minutes. Some doctors will ask you to perform this exploration of fetal movement two times a day. If you're carrying triplets or quads, this may be more difficult, but you may still wish to determine a "baseline" of movement and monitor it.

"Feeling those babies inside me!" Zoe says wistfully. "That's the only part of pregnancy I really miss."

Group B Streptococcus

Around Week 35, your doctor will want to test you for Group B streptococcus, a type of infection that babies can acquire during their passage through the birth canal, leading to the early onset of Group B strep infection in newborns. To avoid this, your cervix, vagina, and rectum will be tested for Group B strep, which you may be carrying without any symptoms. If any of these areas are "colonized" by streptococci, you'll be treated with antibiotics in labor. Premature babies are, as a group, at higher risk for Group B strep, and if you do go into preterm labor, your doctor will test you for Group B strep and then treat you with antibiotics, just in case, until the results of your test are back. Meanwhile, efforts continue to develop a vaccine against Group B strep that could eventually make both testing and treatment unnecessary.

How Your Babies Are Developing

Although your babies will benefit from a longer stay in the womb, Week 24 is when they become potentially viable outside it. If they're born during Week 28, they actually have a 90 percent chance of survival.

If they do stay in the womb, their weight increases significantly during this stage: By Week 28, they'll weigh up to three pounds and measure up to 15 inches long. More fat is developing beneath their skins, and their skins have more pigment. Their hair is growing, their facial features become more distinct, and they are able to open and

Cord Blood: To Harvest or Not to Harvest?

You may already have heard from one of the many agencies offering their services in banking the blood from your babies' umbilical cords. In recent years, much research has been done on stem cells from the placenta, which can regenerate blood in ways similar to bone marrow. So it may be useful to save cord blood, which contains stem cells and which might be used to treat blood disorders such as leukemia as well as some hereditary deficiencies. It may be difficult to match placental stem cells with those of a donor, so the theory is that saving your babies' cord blood might save them the trouble of seeking a donor later on. Also such cells may be useful for siblings.

There are a number of problems with this idea, however. First, it's possible that if a child develops a severe blood disease early on, especially a blood-related cancer, his or her own blood would not be used for a transfusion: If the blood disease has genetic roots, there may be a similar problem in the cord blood.

Second, it's unclear whether blood that's been frozen for many years is still viable for donations. Third, many companies that once offered this service have since gone out of business—after collecting fees from the parents—with no controls over what happens to the blood.

Finally, many people object to the privatization of this service. It costs about $1,500 initially—possibly more for multiples—plus $100 per year thereafter, and it is not covered by most insurance policies. In addition, some doctors charge extra for harvesting blood at the time of delivery. So rather than this private approach, many people prefer the idea of public banking of stem cells, which is being done and which would make stem cells available to anyone who needs them. While there's always the risk of not finding a match, the more people who participate, the better the system works.

I personally think there are better ways of spending $1,500 than on private cord-blood banking, and I advise you not to feel pressured or guilty if you decide not to bank. If you do decide to bank your children's cord blood, the third trimester is the time to make arrangements with a company and with your doctor.

close their eyes, which seems to evidence rapid eye movement (REM), associated with the dreaming stage of sleep. In fact, your babies have their own sleep-wake cycles. Although it's too dark in the womb for them to see anything, they are able to respond to sound by Week 26.

By Week 32, your twins will probably weigh four pounds each—a similar weight to singletons at the same period. Their length is also similar—25 to 40 centimeters. In the second-to-the-last month, your babies' bodies will start to grow somewhat larger in relation to their heads. Except for their lungs, all their organs are working.

The last four or five weeks are especially dramatic. Even though twins, triplets, and quads gain weight a bit more slowly than singletons at this time—otherwise, there wouldn't be room inside you!—your twins will grow from 1,800 to 2,500 grams, or from about 3½ to 5 pounds. A baby usually has to weigh 2,000 grams—over 4 pounds— before being discharged from the hospital, so if your twins are born during Week 32, they'll probably need to spend some time in the intensive-care unit.

During this last month, your twins will grow from 40 to 45 centimeters. They'll start to show more sophisticated motor development, and their lung development really takes off. The lungs' alveolar cells begin to produce surfactant and phospholipids, which help the babies' lungs expand.

13.

If Something Goes Wrong: Complications

⚜

In the multiple-pregnancy balancing act we've been describing, it's important to expect the best—while being prepared for the worst. The complications described in this chapter are concerns that you and your doctor will watch out for. But it's important to remember that *most* pregnancies—even most multiple pregnancies—are free of them. And even when a problem does arise, there are often many ways to manage it.

Diabetes

At some point during your pregnancy, you may feel as though you are constantly hungry—or you may feel fine one moment and starving the next. These experiences of constant or sudden hunger reflect changes in your body's blood sugar.

These changes are a normal part of pregnancy. If you have diabetes, however, whether *chronic/pregestational* (a condition that existed before the pregnancy) or *gestational* (a condition apparently triggered by the pregnancy), your blood-sugar level becomes a greater concern.

Diabetes is a condition in which the body doesn't manufacture enough insulin to metabolize *glucose,* or blood sugar. If you don't have diabetes, there is a delicate balance between insulin, blood sugar, and hunger. You eat, flooding your blood with glucose, which triggers the production of insulin. In about two hours, the insulin has "used up" the glucose, your blood-sugar levels are down, and gradually you experience the sensation of hunger. You respond to the sensation by eating—and the whole process starts all over again. If you have diabetes, however, whether chronic or gestational, your body isn't producing enough insulin to metabolize all that blood sugar or is relatively resistant to its effect.

If you have chronic or pregestational diabetes, you are already aware of your condition, and, ideally, you've been eating right and managing blood sugars from before you started trying to get pregnant. Although diabetics face a risk of bearing children with structural problems that is four times higher than that of the general population, diabetic women who control their blood sugars during pregnancy can lower their risk to basically the same as that of the general population—an empowering thought, and a true incentive to manage your sugars well even before conception.

If you didn't have diabetes when you got pregnant, your doctor should screen you for gestational diabetes. Both conditions pose risks for pregnancy, but some of the risks are different.

Gestational diabetes is especially common in multiple pregnancies. The placental hormones create an environment that favors a diabetic state and increases blood-sugar levels. These hormones exist in even higher levels when the woman is carrying multiples. So if you already had a tendency to diabetes (and especially if you were obese when you got pregnant), the hormones released during your multiple pregnancy might push your body chemistry "over the edge."

My patient Vanessa developed gestational diabetes during her first trimester. "I couldn't believe it," she recalls. "I had always been healthy—maybe a little heavy for my height, but my blood pressure had always been fine, and I was strong. Diabetes seemed like a *very* serious disease, and I couldn't get used to the idea that now I had to take care of myself in a whole new way."

Fortunately, Vanessa's diabetes did not require treatment with insulin. I worked with her to develop a low-carbohydrate diet and went over the basic dietary principles with her—eating regularly, avoiding sweets and processed flour, and monitoring her glucose levels. She had a little trouble sticking to the diet at first. "I'd always been a big bread and pasta person," she points out, "and now that I was pregnant, I was *starving* all the time." Eventually, though, she settled into the swing of things and started working with a nutritionist—and we were able to get her blood sugars under control.

Managing Your Diabetes After the Babies Are Born

Although gestational diabetes usually disappears as soon as the babies are born, about 50 percent of all women who had gestational diabetes may develop overt diabetes within 20 years of their pregnancy. As you can see, follow-up will be very important in the years to come.

Likewise, if you have chronic diabetes, the placental hormones of pregnancy can increase your risk of postpartum complications, especially ophthalmic (relating to the eyes). With good control no worsening of kidney function has been shown, however.

WHO'S AT RISK? Although any pregnant woman can develop gestational diabetes, there are some special risk factors:

- obesity (weighing at least 25 percent more than your ideal weight);
- previous history of gestational diabetes;
- previous infant weighing nine pounds or more (suggesting that there was an undiagnosed condition of gestational diabetes, which tends to produce fatter babies, since the higher fetal insulin levels can act as a growth factor);
- previous unexplained death of a fetus (which might have been caused by diabetes-related problems);
- previous infant with congenital anomaly (because there is an association of chronic diabetes with birth defects);
- family members with diabetes;

- mother over age 25;
- mother currently spilling a lot of sugar into her urine;
- mother in high-risk group such as Native American or Latina.

As it happens, Vanessa didn't fit any of these risk factors. Although she'd weighed a bit more than her ideal when she got pregnant, she was by no means obese. Diabetes didn't run in her family; this was her first pregnancy; and she was only 24. Her condition reminded me that risk factors are really just probabilities—ideas about who *might* become sick. Many women never develop the condition they're supposedly at risk for, while many others suffer from unpredictable problems.

HOW DO YOU KNOW? As we saw in Chapter 10, you will be getting a urine test at every monthly checkup, and your doctor will follow the results closely. Although some glucose in your urine is normal during pregnancy, your doctor will be alerted if your urine continues to show unusually high glucose levels.

There's been a lot of recent debate about whom should be screened for gestational diabetes. Should all pregnant women be tested for this condition, or only those who have special risk factors—obesity and/or a family history of diabetes? As it happens, the "special risk" factors for gestational diabetes aren't very good predictors. (They certainly weren't in Vanessa's case!)

Ethnicity is a slightly better predictor of who's at risk: some 5 to 6 percent of Latina women develop gestational diabetes, versus only 1.4 percent of the general population. And rates among some Native Americans are so high that it may be appropriate to proceed to a full glucose tolerance test (see page 183). But as you can see, if we tested only "at-risk" women, we'd miss some 43 percent of all cases of gestational diabetes.

As with everything else in medicine, the pendulum tends to swing back and forth. The latest standard of care calls for testing *all* pregnant women for gestational diabetes, with high-risk women being screened in their first trimester and other women being screened in the third trimester, when the hormones of pregnancy are most likely to trigger diabetes.

Screening takes the form of a *glucose challenge test*. If you're not obese and have no family history of diabetes, you'll probably be tested sometime between Week 24 and Week 28, which is the time when your insulin reactivity is at its peak. (If you began pregnancy with the high-risk factors just detailed or are severely overweight, if you've had gestational diabetes before, or if you've got a family history of diabetes, you should have been given this test at your diagnostic visit and will then get it again between Week 24 and Week 28.) You'll be asked to drink an extremely sweet solution that contains 50 grams of glucose, and your blood will be tested one hour later. If the glucose levels in your blood are within the standard range (below 140 mg/dl), then you're producing enough insulin to metabolize blood sugar effectively.

Some 10 to 15 percent of the women who take this glucose challenge test will test positive for diabetes—although in fact only 20 to 40 percent of the women who test positive will actually *have* the condition. So if you "fail" the first test, don't worry. You'll be getting a second test that you have an 80 percent chance of "passing": the *glucose tolerance test.*

This second test requires you to fast on the day of the test, and then have a blood sample taken. You are then given 100 grams of another sweet drink, followed by blood tests after one, two, and three hours. The four blood tests—which measure your body's ability to metabolize glucose—reveal whether or not you have gestational diabetes.

HOW WILL GESTATIONAL DIABETES AFFECT YOUR BABIES? The same placental hormones that create the tendency to diabetes also seem to produce heavier babies with larger upper bodies: The fetuses' higher insulin levels seem to work as a growth factor for the babies. You may find this a particular problem if you're carrying not one but two or more heavy fetuses. Although it's a good thing for babies to gain weight in the womb, too *much* weight gain makes it harder for you to carry them to term—and harder to deliver!

Despite Vanessa's good work in controlling her blood sugars, she delivered two 7½-pound babies—a high weight for twins. But the delivery went smoothly, and both of Vanessa's babies were healthy and beautiful.

Gestational diabetes may also cause some fetuses' lungs to mature more slowly than normal, although there is no additional risk of birth defects. Another possible problem is *polyhydramnios,* an excess of fluid in the womb, which further increases the weight you're carrying around and puts you at increased risk for preterm labor as well. (For more on the relationship between gestational diabetes and preterm labor, see Chapter 14.) Moreover, the newborns of a mother with gestational diabetes are at risk for various metabolic disorders, such as problems with blood calcium levels, hypoglycemia, and other conditions. Finally, women with gestational diabetes are at a higher risk of stillbirth. However, as Vanessa found out, *all* of these risks decrease almost to normal with excellent blood-sugar control. (For more on how to manage your blood sugar, see "What You Can Do," below.)

HOW WILL CHRONIC DIABETES AFFECT YOUR BABIES? We have seen that without good control the rate of anomalies is four times higher. If you had diabetes before you became pregnant, your babies may have a tendency to have delayed growth.

This may be because diabetes interferes with the circulation of the blood. Multiples alone can put an extra strain on the placenta too. So if you're a multiple mom with chronic diabetes and a poor supply of blood to your placenta, your babies may be undernourished and their growth may be restricted. There is also a 5 to 10 percent higher risk of preeclampsia and hypertension, for which multiple moms are also at higher risk.

It also seems that the children of women with chronic diabetes can't tolerate labor as well. And, if your blood sugars are not well-controlled, you face a higher risk of stillbirth, which is why close monitoring and fetal surveillance are necessary.

However, all of the risks I've just outlined can be brought down to almost-normal levels if your own blood-sugar levels are well-controlled throughout your pregnancy. If you have chronic diabetes, you probably already know a great deal about how to control your blood sugars. For more suggestions, read on. One problem you *don't* have to worry about is your twins being born with diabetes. If there is a family history of diabetes, they might develop the disease in later life, but they won't be born with it. However, babies sometimes respond to their mother's extra-high levels of glucose with their own extra insulin production, so your doctor will need to make sure that your newborns' glucose levels are carefully monitored.

WHAT YOU CAN DO. Whether you have chronic or gestational diabetes, your goal is to maintain *euglycemia*—even levels of blood sugar. If you've got chronic diabetes, you may already be taking insulin supplements, and your doctor may adjust these in response to the additional demands of pregnancy. During pregnancy, you may need to monitor your glucose levels as often as six to eight times a day. Your goal is to have even better blood-sugar control and more accurate insulin monitoring than normal. Glucose should be (in mg/dl): 60 to 105—fasting; below 140—one hour after meals; below 120—two hours after meals.

If you've got gestational diabetes, your doctor will probably try to avoid insulin injections by encouraging you to eat carefully and exercise regularly, as the demands of your multiple pregnancy permit. However, sometimes insulin *is* necessary, even several times daily. Oral hypoglycemics are never used, and pumps are only rarely used.

With either type of diabetes, you may be given insulin via an IV drip during labor, to help you maintain even levels of blood sugar during the several hours when you won't be able to eat, so that the babies maintain normal glucose levels at birth and in the nursery.

No one should *ever* try to lose weight while pregnant—and that is especially true for women carrying multiples with either kind of diabetes, for whom controlling blood sugars should be their main concern. You might want to consider other ways of controlling your weight after the pregnancy is over, but while you are pregnant, work with your doctor to develop a healthy diet, rich in protein and small amounts of complex carbohydrates (whole grains, whole-grain breads) and low in simple sugars and in foods that have been sweetened or processed. You might want to keep a food journal, scrupulously recording everything you eat and drink, so that you and your doctor can analyze how your diet is affecting your blood sugar as well as your weight. Your doctor will probably also suggest regular, moderate exercise—in keeping with the needs of your multiple pregnancy, of course. (I urged Vanessa to find some kind of physical activity, and she chose swimming. She came to like the exercise so much that she kept it up even after the babies were born!)

Here are some other specific tips:

- **Nutritionists with a special interest in diabetes can be very helpful.** If you have any concern about how to manage your blood sugars while pregnant, see about getting more specific nutritional support.

- **Don't go more than four or five hours without eating, and never skip a meal.** When you miss a meal, your blood sugar goes way down, and you need to eat a great deal to bring it back to normal. This extra eating can in turn set off extra insulin production to metabolize the extra blood sugar—and your levels unbalance again. Three meals plus three snacks a day at fairly regular intervals will help keep your blood-sugar levels nice and even.

- **Avoid sweetened foods—even "naturally" sweet foods.** Fruit juices, fruit-sweetened foods (such as all-fruit jellies), and dried fruits (raisins, figs, prunes, dried apricots) are all extremely high in glucose—and can all increase your blood sugars.

- **Stay away from processed cereals.** You may have felt that your morning bowl of Grape-Nuts or cornflakes was a relatively healthy way to start the day, but most commercial cereals aren't made with whole grains. Switch to a whole-grain cereal—oatmeal, cream of rye, cream of rice—or a whole-grain bread, and limit your carb intake. Sorry: Granola, even the most natural kind, is too sweet for this diet.

- **Eat a high-protein breakfast.** Along with your whole-grain bread or cereal, be sure to eat some protein, which will keep the carbohydrates from pushing your blood sugar up too quickly. Eggs, hard cheese, cottage cheese, lean meat, or fish are all good breakfast foods.

- **Avoid both "open" and "hidden" sweets.** You already know that cakes, candies, pastries, pies, ice cream, frozen yogurt, and other frozen desserts should be avoided. But be on the lookout for hidden sweets, which have been added to virtually all prepared food in the form of sugar, corn syrup, corn sweeteners, honey, molasses, dextrose, fructose (fruit sugars), and glucose. Deceptive sweet foods include granola, canned fruits, baked beans, honey mustard, teriyaki sauce, ketchup, canned or bottled spaghetti sauce, and nondairy creamer.

- **Keep a diet log.** This will help you and your doctor and/or nutritionist figure out what in your diet is working and what isn't, especially on the days when your sugars are high.

Of course, if you have either gestational or chronic diabetes, your doctor will want to keep an especially close watch over your health and that of your babies and will probably start giving you nonstress tests and/or biophysical profiles at between 28 and 36 weeks, depending on the degree of risk present, testing later if the condition is well controlled. (In a nonstress test, you'll be asked to lie down in the doctor's office and record fetal movements by pushing a button on a monitor each time you notice a movement. Ideally, there will be two or more fetal heart rate accelerations in 20 minutes, each lasting at least 15 seconds. Babies who aren't lively enough are monitored further.) Your doctor will also be monitoring your babies closely with regular sonograms, taking regular biophysical profiles to monitor muscle tone, breathing, and other indications of good fetal health.

During labor, your glucose levels will be checked regularly, and you might even have an insulin drip to help control your blood sugars. Your doctor will be concerned to keep your babies from developing hypo- or hyperglycemia and abnormal calcium or bilirubin levels at birth.

Anemia

Nearly 20 percent of all pregnant women become anemic—usually because of low iron levels in the blood. Dilutional anemia occurs when the number of red blood cells is too low relative to the total volume of blood. A woman with a multiple pregnancy has to be especially careful, since her blood volume has vastly increased—up to 100 percent higher than normal. That's why women carrying twins develop anemia 2.4 times more often than women with singletons. Since multiple pregnancies pose a greater risk of hemorrhage, it's especially important to keep your hemoglobin up.

On your diagnostic visit, your doctor will probably check your blood count (the number of red blood cells in a given amount of blood), but you may develop anemia later in the pregnancy.

Frequently, women develop problems sometime around Week 20. As we saw in Chapter 10, your doctor may be checking your hemoglobin levels each trimester.

WHO'S AT RISK? Any pregnant woman can become anemic, and carrying multiple fetuses puts you at special risk. Here are some other risk factors:

- having several babies in a short time;
- vomiting a lot and/or eating little because of morning sickness (as we saw in Chapter 7, multiple moms are at special risk here too);
- beginning the pregnancy in a state of poor nourishment;
- eating poorly throughout the pregnancy;
- beginning the pregnancy with another type of anemia, such as sickle-cell or thalassemia.

HOW DO YOU KNOW? Unfortunately, there are usually no symptoms for pregnancy-related anemia, although some women notice paleness, extreme fatigue, unusual breathlessness, palpitations (a sense of trembling in the chest), or fainting spells. However, any woman carrying multiples might expect extreme fatigue and, as we've seen in Chapter 10, breathlessness as well, so regular blood testing is your only way to be sure.

HOW WILL YOUR BABIES BE AFFECTED? This is one of the few cases in which the babies' nutritional needs are met before the mother's, since when mildly anemic women give birth, their babies seem to have normal iron levels. However, severely anemic women tend to give birth prematurely and to deliver babies at somewhat lower birth weights.

WHAT CAN YOU DO? As we saw in Chapter 7, eating a diet rich in iron and taking some iron supplements is your best protection against anemia. Deficiencies of folic acid and vitamin B_{12} may cause anemia as well—but most prenatal vitamins include these, along with a small amount (30–60 mg) of iron. Work with your doctor to find the right level of supplementation while eating high-fiber foods and drinking lots of water to prevent iron-related constipation. If signs of anemia persist, your doctor might want to test you for another type of anemia, such as sickle-cell or thalassemia. (For more on folic acid, see Chapter 7. For more on sickle-cell and thalassemia, see Chapter 2.) He or she will also check your iron levels and your ability to create new red blood cells.

Preeclampsia and Hypertension

Eclampsia is a term for seizures that result from high blood pressure. *Preeclampsia* is the condition that leads to eclampsia. Preeclampsia management, therefore, is intended to prevent the onset of eclampsia.

There are three types of pregnancy-induced hypertension (PIH): hypertension alone, that associated with preeclampsia, and that associated with eclampsia. Some 37 percent of all mothers of twins and 46 percent of all mothers of triplets suffer from pregnancy-induced hypertension (a blood-pressure reading higher than 140 over 90). So one major goal of pregnancy management is to monitor women with PIH so that we can diagnose preeclampsia as early as possible.

Edema is also very common: Some one-third of all pregnant women suffer from edema by their 38th week. However, the edema associated with preeclampsia is usually worse: The hands and face swell up, rings feel tight, and the swelling is present even first thing in the morning. Since the "classic triad" of preeclampsia is hypertension (high blood pressure), edema (swelling), and proteinuria (protein in the urine), if your doctor suspects that your edema is related to preeclampsia, he or she will take your blood pressure and test the protein in your urine. A count of more than 300 mg of protein in a urine sample is an indication of a possible problem.

Even when proteinuria is *not* associated with preeclampsia, it carries a higher risk for newborns and mothers. The risk goes up further when proteinuria is associated with PIH, and even further when it's associated with preeclampsia.

My patient Rosario developed PIH, and I was very concerned to keep it from turning into preeclampsia. Rosario had a history of difficulty with elevated blood pressure even before she got pregnant, in addition to being about 20 pounds overweight. We monitored her blood pressure and urine closely and kept a close watch on signs of edema.

WHO'S AT RISK? Women most at risk for preeclampsia are those who began their pregnancies with chronic high blood pressure and/or diabetes and women in their first pregnancies. Women pregnant with multiples are at particular risk as well.

HOW DO YOU KNOW? It's perfectly possible to have preeclampsia without any symptoms except for a high reading on your blood-pressure test and the indications of protein in your urine. Symptoms that you might notice without tests include a sudden weight gain that doesn't seem to be related to an increased intake of food; severe swelling of hands and face; unexplained headaches or itching; and disturbances of vision.

Liver Problems and Preeclampsia

Your doctor will be monitoring your liver function closely, as there are some rare liver malfunctions associated with preeclampsia. One of these is the so-called fatty liver of pregnancy, in which the liver has difficulty metabolizing fat. A slightly more common condition is HELLP (Hemolysis, Elevated Liver [enzymes], and Low Platelets), which involves disturbed liver function and affects the platelet and blood counts. These are serious conditions, and they often require doctors to deliver promptly.

WHAT CAN YOU DO? Your doctor will be giving you regular urine and blood-pressure checks on your monthly office visits, so any problems with increased blood pressure or extra protein in your urine should show up then. It's rare for preeclampsia to appear before Week 20.

Since preeclampsia is a risk factor for preterm labor, your doctor will be engaged in a balancing act: prolonging your pregnancy while ensuring your health and safety. In many cases, home bed rest is the first step in treatment, as your doctor continues to monitor your blood pressure and the health of your fetuses. (For more about bed rest, see Chapter 9.) In more severe cases, your doctor may decide to hospitalize you and/or deliver, either by inducing labor for a vaginal birth or by performing a cesarean. The choice of delivery method will depend on your condition, your babies' condition, their gestational age, and their position and weight. Either way, if you're between 24 and 36 weeks, your doctor may try to postpone the delivery for 48 hours, while your babies are given steroids to speed up the maturation of their lungs—assuming that your condition permits the delay.

Of course, your doctor will be monitoring you closely for complications, such as platelet abnormalities or changes in your liver function. You'll also be getting sonograms and nonstress tests to make sure that your babies are growing well and getting an adequate blood supply.

Magnesium sulfate is given intravenously to prevent seizures, a treatment that also tends to lower your blood pressure. If your blood pressure is very high, your doctor may want to give you other medications to bring it down and to prevent possible serious complications, such as stroke. You will be monitored closely postpartum, and your doctor may continue to give you magnesium sulfate for the next 24 hours after delivery.

The Loss of a Twin

The loss of one baby in a multiple pregnancy is remarkably common. As we've seen, most losses take place in the first trimester, with an excellent prognosis for the surviving fetus.

After the first trimester, there's a 2 to 5 percent chance that one twin will die, a figure that is even higher for monochorionic twins. Many times, the lost twin suffered from some kind of structural abnormality that might have prevented the child from surviving after birth. Some 15 percent of all triplet pregnancies also result in the loss of one of the triplets.

If a twin is lost in the second or third trimester, there may be a 30 percent mortality rate for the surviving twin. Again, the problems—both the mortality rates and the neurological defects—tend to be far higher among monochorionic twins. There's been some speculation that this is because monochorionic twins have more "vascular communication"—that is, they share blood vessels running through the placenta. Thus clots or other problems in those communicating vessels may lead to a decrease in blood supply, which in turn causes complications for the survivor. However, delivering a surviving monochorionic baby immediately after the death of its twin does not seem to affect the loss rate among survivors, so if extreme prematurity is a factor, waiting to deliver may be prudent.

Once the surviving baby's lungs have matured, the doctor will want to deliver quickly. A vaginal delivery might still be possible. With dizygotic twins, there's less risk associated with waiting. At the time of delivery, your doctor might see a flattened fetus in the fetal membranes known as fetus papyraceus.

Intrauterine Growth Restriction

Intrauterine growth restriction (IUGR), also known as *intrauterine growth retardation,* is a condition in which fetuses don't grow at the appropriate rate. While the condition occurs in only 5 to 7 percent of all singleton pregnancies, it marks up to 29 percent of all twin gestations. Twins who have suffered from IUGR face a mortality rate that is 2.5 times higher than that of twins who grew normally. Recent epidemiological data shows that abnormal fetal growth may even be associated with increased risk of cardiovascular disease or diabetes later in life—a kind of in utero programming! Usually, however, IUGR affects only one of the twins in the pair.

One of the reasons I recommend regular sonograms is so that the doctor can closely monitor the growth of the fetuses and identify IUGR as soon as it occurs. If one or more fetuses seems to weigh below the 10th percentile of what's expected, or if there's a difference of more than 20 percent between the twins (20 percent of the larger twin's weight), then we usually diagnose IUGR.

The American College of Obstetricians and Gynecologists (ACOG) recommends assessing twin growth with special growth tables specifically relating to multiple pregnancies. These tables show that twins and singletons should grow at the same rate during the first two trimesters but that twin growth flattens considerably in the third trimester. However, this flattening doesn't occur until the very end of the pregnancy: A recent study of almost 20,000 normal twins and singletons found that twins didn't begin to differ in their growth patterns until after Week 30. Twins' low fetal growth rates might once have been considered normal, but now we know that they may be suffering either from IUGR or from an inability of the placenta(s) to adequately nourish both fetuses.

If your doctor suspects that your babies are suffering from this syndrome, he or she will want to monitor their progress closely. While dichorionic twins probably need only monthly sonograms, mono-chorionic twins should be monitored every two to three weeks after Week 24. Your doctor will also be giving you frequent nonstress tests and/or biophysical profiles to make sure that your babies are thriving. If they're not, your doctor may decide to induce delivery early.

When my patient Pat had her regular monthly sonogram in her sixth month, I noticed that her babies did not seem to be growing as quickly as they should. Since her twins were monochorionic, I had al-ready scheduled biweekly sonograms for her. I suggested that she be extra careful about getting enough nutrients and asked her to cut back on her usual vigorous schedule of exercise. The sonograms continued to show unusually slow growth, and I became more concerned. After a couple of weeks of bed rest, the twins had good internal growth but they still remained in the bottom 10th percentile for their gestational age. So at 33 weeks, we tested Pat's amniotic fluid and then gave Pat steroids to help her babies' lungs mature. After another sonogram showed breech presentation, we delivered Pat by C-section. Her ba-bies weighed just over three pounds each—a cause for some con-cern—but they soon began to put on weight and to thrive.

HIV

I can't stress it too strongly: Every pregnant woman should be screened for HIV. Many women feel that they're not at risk for HIV, because they don't fit the profile of the most at-risk groups. But it's been well established that women outside these high-risk groups can also have HIV—and they're putting their unborn children at high risk if the HIV goes undetected.

If you're screened for HIV and you test positive, there *is* pregnancy-related treatment that can vastly reduce the chance of transmitting the virus to your fetuses. You can be treated in the third trimester and during labor. You also need to avoid breast-feeding, since breast milk can transmit the virus.

New York state law now mandates testing all babies whose moth-ers do not have test results on their prenatal charts, and other states seem to be passing similar legislation. Whether or not to be tested is a decision that you alone can make—but I'd advise in favor. HIV screening can be done as part of a routine blood test.

Rh Incompatibility

Another common prenatal complication is Rh incompatibility. To oversimplify a bit, we might say that every human being is born either Rh positive (with blood that includes the Rh factor) or Rh negative (without that factor). If you're one of the 85 percent of all human beings who are Rh positive, you have no cause for concern. Or if you and the baby's father are both Rh negative, there's no problem either.

However, if you are Rh negative and your baby's father is Rh positive, there's a chance that your baby could inherit the father's Rh-positive factor. And when your baby's blood cells enter your blood, your body will develop an immune response, producing antibodies to "protect" you from this "foreign" substance.

Usually, this isn't a problem in a first pregnancy. If this is *not* your first pregnancy, however, and if one or both of your twins is Rh positive, the antibodies still in your system might cross the placenta and attack your babies' red blood cells. One or both of your babies could develop mild to severe anemia and, in more severe cases, heart failure and a condition known as *hydrops fetalis*—a generalized swelling of the fetus and the accumulation of fluid around all the fetal cavities and organs.

Rh incompatibility used to be a far greater danger than it is today. Now, however, we have developed Rh-immune globulin, a substance that can prevent the development of Rh-negative antibodies. This substance is usually given at least twice, unless the father is known to be Rh negative:

- In Week 28, an Rh-negative woman who shows no antibodies in her blood is given a dose of Rh-immune globulin.
- After delivery (or after miscarriage, abortion, or bleeding during second and third trimesters of pregnancy), another dose is administered.
- Within 72 hours after invasive procedures such as CVS or am-

niocentesis or even external cephalic version (turning a breech baby), a dose is given.

If you're Rh negative, it's important to remember that you might have developed antibodies during an ectopic pregnancy or a pregnancy that miscarried. A particularly heavy menstrual period might indicate an undiagnosed early miscarriage—in which some fetal blood cells entered your circulatory system. In other words, if you're Rh negative with an Rh-positive partner, and there's *any* chance you've been pregnant before, you need to take RhoGAM, the Rh-immune globulin.

If you *have* developed antibodies, in this or a previous pregnancy, your doctor will monitor your antibody levels regularly. If these levels rise, the doctor will go on to assess your babies' condition. Amniocentesis can reveal whether your twins are suffering from a breakdown of blood cells measured by the amount of bilirubin pigment. If so, the specialist may puncture the babies' umbilical cord and take a sample of their blood. That test should reveal whether one or both babies is anemic, in which case they'll be given a fetal blood transfusion. Thanks to RhoGAM, however, transfusions are needed in fewer than one percent of all Rh-incompatible pregnancies.

There are also rare red-cell antigens in some Rh groups, a few of which may cause blood diseases for newborns. On your first prenatal visit, your doctor will screen for these rare antibodies once your blood type is determined.

Special Risks

As we saw in Chapter 3, monozygotic twins who share a chorion are at special risk of certain conditions. This is another reason for your doctor to use sonography to assess what type of twins you're carrying, so you'll be aware of the risks.

TWIN–TWIN TRANSFUSION SYNDROME. Monochorionic twins sometimes have a condition in which blood from one twin literally flows into the other, creating a "donor" and a "recipient" twin.

Although almost all monochorionic twins have some vascular communication, it poses a problem for only about 15 percent of all monochorionic twins, or for 5 to 10 percent of all twins. Connections between one twin's arteries and the other one's veins are the riskiest.

In extreme cases, the condition poses risks to both donor and recipient. The donor twin becomes anemic, has little or no amniotic fluid, and grows at a slower rate, so that he or she weighs at least 20 percent less than the other twin. He or she may also appear to be "stuck" to the uterine wall. The recipient twin is not much better off: He or she is polycythemic—having too *much* blood—and oversized. The recipient twin is also likely to produce a great deal of amniotic fluid, which puts some 10 to 25 percent of recipient twins at risk of congestive heart failure.

This syndrome usually emerges sometime between Week 16 and Week 26, although it may not be possible for your doctor to spot it until Weeks 20 through 30. About 95 percent of the time, both twins are structurally normal. However, the other 5 percent of the time, fetal anomalies are associated with the condition. The condition may also be associated with *placental insufficiency,* in which the placenta is not providing the twins with sufficient nourishment or oxygen.

Over 70 percent of twin–twin transfusion cases go untreated, mainly because the syndrome is so hard to detect. Untreated, though, this condition can be serious.

Treatment depends on when the condition is diagnosed. If it shows up late in the pregnancy, your doctor will probably try to deliver you as soon as possible. If your babies are too young for this response, your doctor may perform amniocentesis to remove some of the excess amniotic fluid from the recipient twin's sac. There are other more experimental treatments that involve such methods as using lasers to stop blood from flowing through the vessels connecting the twins. Your doctor can tell you about the latest information on treatments for this condition.

MONOAMNIOTIC TWINS. Although only 1 percent of all monozygotic twins are monoamniotic (see Chapter 3), this is an extremely high-risk category, with a 50 percent fetal mortality rate. Naturally, we want to make an early diagnosis of the condition and keep both mother and babies under close surveillance. Because the chances of fetal mortality are so high, some women even choose to terminate this type of pregnancy. The condition can be diagnosed by sonogram, usually late in the first trimester or early in the second trimester, when the sonogram reveals that there is no membrane separating the two fetuses. The sonogram may also show that the babies' cords are entangled—a clear sign that they're monoamniotic and an indication that they can have up to a 70 percent chance of fetal death.

As you can see, a monoamniotic pregnancy requires intense supervision, which each doctor will tailor to the needs of his or her patients. If you're pregnant with monoamniotic twins, expect frequent nonstress tests and sonograms to assess your twins' size and to keep updating their biophysical profiles. Your doctor will be measuring their tone and breathing rate while keeping track of how much amniotic fluid is in your womb.

The possibility of entangled cords makes a vaginal delivery extremely unwise for monoamniotic twins. It's also difficult to know which twin's cord to clamp as the first baby is delivered.

I recall one of my patients, Luz, who was pregnant with monoamniotic twins. We treated her babies with steroids at 32 weeks to give their lungs an extra boost and then delivered her by C-section. Both of her babies came out healthy and strong—which to me ranked as one of the near-miracles that modern science makes possible.

CONJOINED TWINS. The inaccurate—and racially biased—popular term for this condition is "Siamese twins," in which twins share organs and other structures. This type of complication—although fascinating—is extraordinarily rare. Despite its popularity in legend, this condition is found in only 1 of 50,000 births. The condition is suspected when the sonogram doesn't seem to allow the twins to be visualized separately. It's possible that parents of conjoined twins would choose to terminate the pregnancy. If not, ideally, the babies would be delivered as early as possible—by 26 weeks, in most cases—by means of a C-section.

ACARDIAC TWINNING. This is another extremely rare condition that's more of a medical curiosity than an actual possibility. An acardiac twin has no cranium (skull), thorax (midsection), or heart, yet manages to sustain life through the blood flow of the normal twin. This condition puts the twin with the heart at a greater than 50 percent risk of death, and preterm delivery is common as well. Recent research suggests that the best way to increase the chances for the normal twin to survive is to ligate the umbilical cord of the acardiac twin, who will not be able to survive out of the womb, which can even be done laparoscopically.

14.

Avoiding Preterm Labor and Premature Birth

&c—&co

All women carrying twins or higher-order multiples face an increased risk of preterm labor and the delivery of premature babies. But some women are at higher risk than others. In this chapter,
I'll help you understand what causes preterm labor and help you evaluate your risk. In the following chapter, we'll consider options that
can help prevent preterm labor. In Chapter 16, we'll talk about times
when your doctor may actually want to deliver you early.

What Is Preterm Labor?

Preterm labor is the technical term for contractions associated with dilation of the cervix before babies have reached full term, which for
singleton pregnancies is identified as 40 weeks. However, many specialists believe that 37 to 38 weeks may be enough time to carry twins
and other multiples.

Another definition of premature birth is based on weight. Most
doctors consider a baby born at less than 5½ pounds (2,500 grams) to
have been born prematurely. The latter definition is a little less useful
for multiples, though, given that some 53 percent of all twins have low

birth weight. That figure is seven times higher than the 7.4 percent low-birth-weight rate of all U.S. babies.

A third commonly accepted way of thinking about prematurity is that a baby born before 37 weeks is preterm, while one born before 33 weeks is very preterm. A baby born at less than 2,500 grams—5½ pounds—has a low birth weight, while a child born at less than 1,500 grams—3⅓ pounds—has a very low birth weight.

Why is this terminology important? Prematurity and low birth weight are correlated to problems in outcomes, so babies that are very premature and of very low birth weight are more likely to have serious problems.

How Long Should You Carry Your Babies?

Sometimes a woman can't or shouldn't carry her babies to full term. Maybe the babies aren't growing properly, or the mother may have some medical condition that endangers her or her children. So your doctor may decide to induce labor before you've carried to term. Depending on your and your babies' condition, your doctor might also decide to perform a C-section before you've reached full term. (For more on induced labor and early C-sections, see Chapter 16.)

In fact, some data suggests that after 38 weeks, it's better to induce labor than to let twins stay in the womb. Fetuses rely on the placenta for nourishment, and there's some evidence to suggest that placentas in a multiple pregnancy tend not to work as efficiently after the 39th week, putting the babies at risk of not getting the oxygen and nutrients they need. However, other pregnancies continue to flourish well into Weeks 39 and 40—so increased monitoring is probably a better solution than a blanket decision to induce labor. Other factors in this decision are the babies' position (headfirst or feetfirst) and station (how far down they are), as well as how "favorable" your cervix is—that is, how dilated, effaced, and soft it is and what position the cervical opening is in relationship to the first baby's presenting part.

Getting your babies to a reasonable gestational age or close to term is one of the best things you can do for them. Conversely, prematurity is one of the greatest hazards your unborn babies face.

Prematurity is a particular problem for the mothers of twins and other multiples. In this age of advanced medical knowledge, only 9 percent of all singletons are born before the 37th week and less than 2 percent are born before the 31st week. But multiple moms face more sobering statistics. Over half of all twins are born before the 37th week, while over 80 percent of all triplets are born that early. Almost 10 percent of all twins are born before 28 weeks, while more than 20 percent are born before the 31st week.

Of even more concern are the low birth weights that go with these early deliveries. Almost 10 percent of all twins weigh less than 3½ pounds (1,500 grams) at birth, compared to less than 1 percent of all singletons. Of course, it isn't the low birth weight per se that is a concern, but the higher rates of sickness and death that go with it: Preterm babies account for more than 85 percent of all perinatal (birth-related) complications and mortality.

These figures are enough to make a doctor humble, for despite all of the miraculous medical advances of the past 70 years, we have just as high a rate of preterm labor and premature delivery for multiple births now as we did in the 1920s. What we *can* be proud of is the vastly increased survival rate for twins, triplets, quads, and quints. These days, thanks to the advances of medical science, even babies born before the 26th week have a fighting chance to live normal, healthy lives.

Unfortunately, there's still a lot we don't understand about preterm labor. There's no sure way to prevent it, and, if it happens to you, there's not necessarily one best way to cope with it.

What *is* helpful, though, is developing your own personal coping strategy. Even if you can't fully control your risk of preterm labor, you can choose how you will respond to that risk.

I'll never forget my first visit to the hospital room of my patient Monica, for whom I'd had to order bed rest early in her twin pregnancy. I was struck by how thoroughly she had turned the cold, sterile environment of the hospital into her own warm, personal space. A soft quilt in beautiful colors covered the bed; teddy bears, flowers, and photographs of her loved ones adorned the bed table; good-luck cards papered the walls; soothing music flowed from her CD player. Monica would certainly have preferred to be up and about, or at least resting at home. But by making the hospital room her own, she had found a way to make some kind of peace with her situation. She celebrated each day of continued pregnancy as a remarkable achievement—and she delivered two healthy babies at 35 weeks.

What Causes Preterm Labor?

It might be easier to prevent preterm labor if we knew exactly what caused it. Unfortunately, not only do we not know the exact causes of preterm labor, we're not even sure exactly what sets off full-term labor.

However, we do know quite a bit about the biochemical and physiological events that happen as labor approaches, and medical knowledge in this field is advancing all the time. Here's our latest thinking on the subject:

TRIGGERS OF LABOR. The goal of your pregnancy is to keep your fetuses *inside* your uterus. The goal of labor and the birthing process is to get those fetuses *out*. So one way of understanding the triggers of labor is to see them as a release from the inhibiting effects of pregnancy on the uterine muscle.

During pregnancy, the uterus is in a quiet or resting stage, thanks to various hormones—progesterone, relaxin, prostacyclin, and many others. Then, as term approaches, other hormones come into play—estrogen among them—to activate the uterus and prepare for its contractions to be coordinated. The uterus may contract at various points of the pregnancy—occasional contractions known as Braxton-Hicks, for example, are common during the last few weeks of term. But in order for birth to occur, the uterine contractions have to be *coordinated,* and they have to continue over a long period of time. The activation stage is a preparation for these sustained, coordinated contractions.

Once the uterus is activated, it needs to be stimulated. Your body produces two key hormones, oxytocin and prostaglandin, that stimulate the uterus to contract.

What sets off that initial stimulation? Here's where it gets mysterious. Interestingly, we know a lot more about how the process works in sheep and cattle: The maturation of the baby lamb or calf triggers the mother's body to go into labor (which means that prematurity is extremely rare for those species). In humans, though, the process is more complicated and seems to have more to do with a series of changes in the uterus—changes that might, and often do, occur before the fetus(es) are ready to be born.

HORMONAL CHANGES. First, the level of prostaglandins rises. This chemical change produces another change: The uterine muscle cells begin to work together in the coordinated way that will be necessary if they are to produce a long series of contractions. At the same time, these cells develop *oxytocin receptors*—the mechanism by which they can receive the natural hormone oxytocin and thus be affected by oxytocin's tendency to stimulate contractions.

Once the uterus is prepared, it can be affected by factors involving the fetus(es) and placenta—the fetoplacental unit. For example, once the fetoplacental unit reaches a certain size, that might trigger a switch in the uterine muscle activity, creating the regular, coordinated contractions that will help push the fetus(es) out of the womb. (Since size is a factor, the body sometimes misreads an early twin or triplet pregnancy as a singleton pregnancy that is further along. Even in a singleton pregnancy, polyhydramnios—extra fluid in the amniotic sac—can miscue the body to begin labor.)

What other aspects of the fetuses and placenta help trigger labor? One is the hormones that the fetuses release as they mature. Another can be a chemical "mistake": Some 15 percent of preterm labor may be caused by an enzyme deficiency in the fetal membranes that does not allow the breakdown of prostaglandins. (If the prostaglandins remain in their original form, their levels rise—and the process of labor is triggered.)

Another factor is a hostile uterine environment. If there's an infection in the mother's genitals, kidneys, or urinary tract, the fetuses and placenta experience it as a threat. Their response to this threat can help trigger labor.

Infection can also weaken the fetal membranes. If those weakened membranes then rupture, your body reads that as a signal to begin the birth process, even if it's several weeks too early.

A trauma, such as a car accident or a fall, might separate the placenta from the uterine wall—a condition known as *placental abruption*. (For more on placental abruption, see "Additional Risk Factors,"

Cutting-Edge Science: Using Sonograms to Measure the Length of Your Cervix

The condition of your cervix is one very good indicator of how likely you are to give birth. The shorter your cervix, the longer your babies have been in the womb—and the more likely they are to be born. However, sometimes a shorter cervix indicates possible preterm labor. If your cervix length is in the bottom 10 percent for the length of your term, you're six times as likely to deliver before Week 35. If your cervix is abnormally short—say, less than 15 mm at 23 weeks—you've got a 60 percent chance of delivering before 25 weeks and a 90 percent chance of delivering before 32 weeks.

The standard measure of the cervix has traditionally been the pelvic exam. Recent data, though, suggests that a transvaginal sonogram may be a more accurate way of measuring the length of your cervix. That's because part of your cervix may be in your abdomen, to which a standard pelvic exam has no access. A sonogram allows your entire cervix to be measured.

The clinical usefulness of this method is still evolving. But for patients at high risk for preterm delivery—including mothers of multiples—the technique is a valuable addition to our current predictive tools.

Should a multiple mom with no other risk factors for preterm labor be given this test? That's controversial. Some doctors believe the test is useful in any case of multiples. Ultrasound can also be used to check for the funneling of the membranes into the cervical canal, another predictor of possible risk. Other doctors believe that there's no reason to subject every woman to one more costly and invasive exam.

page 215.) A detached placenta may cause thrombin, another hormone, to be released from the uterus, which in turn triggers the uterus to contract. That's why your obstetrician will probably ask you to avoid skiing, horseback riding, and other vigorous sports that put you at risk of a fall.

RISK FACTORS AND MULTIPLE PREGNANCIES. Any pregnancy might end in premature labor. But multiple pregnancies are at par-

Cutting-Edge Science: Fetal Fibronectin Testing

Fetal fibronectin (FFN) is a kind of protein that is found in high levels in the cervix and in vaginal secretions before the onset of labor. If a woman is likely to carry to term, FFN levels are so low between Weeks 18 and 36 that they should not be able to be measured. If your doctor *can* detect FFN in your system, that suggests a higher risk of premature delivery.

The FFN exam is performed between Weeks 24 and 34. It's a simple test: The doctor uses a speculum to roll a swab over your cervix and vagina, making sure not to use any lubricant or antiseptic before the test. The swab is sent to the lab, which can now send results back within an hour. If you test negative—no FFN levels detected—there's an excellent chance that you won't be delivering within the next two weeks and a very good chance that you won't deliver before Week 37.

If you test positive, the results are less certain. However, the FFN test has been able to identify some 64 percent of all women who deliver early, although it may be somewhat less useful for multiple moms. Many doctors recommend FFN testing for multiple moms at 26 weeks. That way, if you test positive, you could consider reducing your workload, possibly get home fetal monitoring (see Chapter 15), and schedule more prenatal visits. And if the test is negative—especially if you've been worried by some infrequent uterine contractions—it can be very reassuring.

ticular risk. First, the pregnancy itself is already a risk factor, because your distended uterus and extra amniotic fluid cause the body to "misread" your pregnancy as further along than it is. Second, certain "extra" risk factors are more associated with multiple pregnancies, such as pregnancy-induced hypertension, polyhydramnios, or an incompetent cervix (a cervix that could manage one baby, for example, might not be able to manage two). So a multiple pregnancy sometimes tends to "multiply" risk factors—and premature labor is the result.

By now you're probably wondering which risk factors *you* have. Take heart: Many of the risk factors for preterm labor can be detected

Cutting-Edge Science: Salivary Estriol Levels

Estriols are a kind of female hormone that were first studied in the 1970s, when they were measured in urine tests. Now they're assessed in saliva—where they've proven to be a useful indicator of the risks of preterm labor.

Estriols in the body rise just before the onset of labor. They help prepare the uterus to coordinate its contractions and, eventually, signal the labor process to begin. About 95 percent of the estriols in a mother's blood are produced by the fetus(es), so estriol levels are another one of those fetoplacental factors that apparently help to trigger labor.

We've discovered that estriol levels tend to surge about three weeks before a preterm birth. They can be measured in the urine, the blood, or in the saliva, but it's easiest to test the saliva. A commercial test is now available.

The test's predictive power is greatest after 30 weeks, and a negative test is more reliable than a positive. In other words, 99 percent of the women who test negative won't deliver within the next week, whereas only some of the women who test positive *will* deliver early. Also, these data apply to *all* mothers: Specific data on twin pregnancies is not yet available. Still, if you're at risk for preterm labor, you might want to discuss the possibility of salivary estriol testing with your doctor.

through your doctor's careful attention to your reproductive history and through routine prenatal exams. Many others show up readily on sonograms. So if you've already had your first prenatal doctor's visit, your doctor has probably ruled out many of the risk factors I'll be discussing in this chapter. Certainly, he or she will stay alert, giving you extra pelvic exams and possibly using some of the many new diagnostic tools that are now available: sonographic measure of cervical length, fetal fibronectin testing, and the measurement of salivary estriol levels.

Coping well with psychological stress can also make a big difference. Of course, that's easier said than done, especially when you're pregnant with twins, but it's a desirable goal nonetheless! After all, you're not just a body carrying two unborn children. You're also a woman who may be working, in a relationship, running a household, maintaining friendships, and keeping up with the other activities that are important to you. The better all these areas of your life are working, the better you'll feel about your pregnancy. And that "feeling better" translates into a greater chance of avoiding the stress that could help trigger preterm labor. (For more on coping with the strains of multiple pregnancy, see Chapter 4.)

"I really think visualization helped," says Natalie. "Every day I'd sit down and imagine my two healthy, beautiful babies, growing as they should, staying inside me for as long as they needed. Of course, I don't know how that affected *them*—but I know it made *me* feel better. And I have to believe that anything that was good for me *was* good for them."

What Are the Risk Factors?

Here's a look at some of the *other* risk factors. The more risk factors on your list, the higher your chances of going into preterm labor. Of course, it goes without saying that your doctor should be informed of each of these factors!

- **Poor nutrition.** Early and adequate weight gain is one of the best ways to protect and nurture your unborn children. Make especially sure you get plenty of protein, lots of milk products, and extra folic acid. (For more on nutrition and diet, see Chapter 7.)
- **Smoking.** This can lead to abruptio placentae and vaginal bleeding, IUGR, and low-birth-weight babies, all of which are associated with preterm delivery.
- **Inadequate hydration.** Athletes know that to perform at their best, they have to drink plenty of water. Although we don't know exactly what the relationship is between hydration and preterm labor, research shows that an irritable uterus and more frequent contractions might be associated with dehydration. I've certainly seen many cases in which a woman's uterus was "irritable"—contracting—until she was adequately hydrated. And

Am I at Risk?: Possible Risk Factors for Preterm Labor

Poor nutrition

Smoking

Inadequate hydration (not enough water in your system)

Emotional stress

Previous premature labor or delivery

Pregnancy-induced hypertension (PIH)

Obesity

Underweight

Congenital anomalies

Chromosomal anomalies

Fibroids

Exposure to ionizing radiation (X rays), anesthetic gases, lead

Auto or bus accident, or other injury

Two or more second-trimester abortions

Diabetes mellitus

Placenta previa

Placental abruption

Problems with hormone production

Genital infections

Kidney and urinary-tract infections

Enzyme deficiencies

Uterine anomalies

Cervical incompetence

Exposure to DES

Oligohydramnios (insufficient amniotic fluid)

Polyhydramnios (excess amniotic fluid)

Premature rupture of membranes (PROM)

multiple moms, with their increased metabolic rate, have a special need to take in enough fluids throughout each day. (For more on hydration, see Chapter 7.)

- **Emotional stress.** There are lots of reasons for feeling stressed out, especially when you're pregnant with multiples. If there's anything about the pregnancy that seems particularly difficult—say, coping without a partner, dealing with a recent move or divorce, facing increased responsibilities at work, or undergoing financial pressures—the stress might increase the risk of preterm labor. That's because your body under stress tends to release extra adrenaline, and adrenaline is a *vasoconstrictor*—it constricts your blood vessels. The consequent reduced blood supply to the uterus might stimulate preterm labor. (For more on using visualization, massage, self-hypnosis, and relaxation exercises to cope with stress, see Chapter 4.)

- **Previous premature labor or delivery.** If you've ever gone into premature labor before, you're at higher risk to do it again. Your previous experience doesn't *cause* future problems. But your history *is* a good predictor of future problems, since whatever caused your first bout with prematurity might continue to affect this pregnancy. My patient Imani, for example, delivered a son at 34 weeks. So when she got pregnant with twins, I wanted her to be very cautious. Although we agreed that she could continue working in her job as a university secretary, I insisted that she find a way to put her feet up and relax completely for 15 minutes in mid-morning, 15 minutes in mid-afternoon, and an hour and a half at lunch. Fortunately, her supervisor allowed her to make the schedule change, although he did insist on reducing her pay. Imani was upset about the loss in income—but agreed that it was preferable to leaving work altogether.

- **Pregnancy-induced hypertension/toxemia (PIH).** This problem is far more common among women carrying twins, which is one of the reasons why twins are more likely than singletons to be premature. Your doctor will be watching you closely for signs of PIH. She or he may treat you with baby aspirin or calcium if you have additional risk factors for preeclampsia, such as chronic hypertension. (For more on PIH and preeclampsia, see Chapter 13.)

- **Obesity.** Obesity is associated with chronic hypertension, pregnancy-induced hypertension, diabetes, and other conditions that in turn are associated with preterm delivery. If you were obese when you got pregnant, or if you had problems with high blood pressure, diabetes, and related conditions, your doctor will be watching you closely. Although it's crucial for you to get good nutrition, your doctor may recommend a different level of weight gain for you than for a woman who started her pregnancy at a lower weight. (For more on nutrition and weight gain, see Chapter 7.)

- **Underweight.** Being underweight doesn't *cause* preterm labor. But if you *are* underweight, you're more likely to have babies with low birth weights. And if you *do* go into preterm labor and deliver early, your low-birth-weight babies will face far greater risks than babies born at higher weights. Twins tend to have a lower birth weight than singletons in any case, which can further exacerbate the problem.

  The classic studies of poor maternal weight gain were conducted in England after World War II. England, recovering from years of wartime, was plagued with food shortages, which meant that expectant mothers were taking in fewer calories—and delivering babies with lower birth weights. These lower birth weights were in turn associated with babies who survived less often or who were less healthy. Low-birth-weight babies, deprived of vital nutrients, might also have suffered from IUGR, or intrauterine growth restriction, in which babies don't thrive in the womb, usually because the placenta isn't sufficient to nourish them properly.

  Nowadays, underweight may be the result of a social problem—a woman is too poor to afford enough good food; a famine keeps everyone from getting enough food. But mothers may also be underweight because they've been dieting strenuously in an attempt to stay thin even while pregnant or because they're bulimic. As we saw, for Shana, the runway model, a svelte figure was essentially a job requirement, so her fear of gaining weight was especially intense. But I've also seen women with no economic reason to stay thin blanch with fear as they approach the scale, stripping off every piece of their clothing, their jewelry, even their wedding rings, to chisel those last few extra ounces off the dreaded total. "I can't believe I'm going to weigh as much as my husband!" Miriam once said to me in despair. "Do I really have to be this big?"

  The answer, in most cases, is yes. Think about it: You're carrying two fetuses, two sacs of amniotic fluid, two placentas. Your breasts are bigger, your uterus is bigger, you're carrying a far larger volume of blood. If you're not eating enough to support that weight gain, you're probably not getting the vitamins, min-

erals, proteins, and other nutrients that you *and* your babies
need to make it through the pregnancy. And poor nutrition—
leading to fetuses who are too small for their age—makes
preterm labor a far more risky business, especially among mothers of twins.

Recent research has shown that women who started their
pregnancies while they were underweight need to gain even
more weight during pregnancy, especially if they're pregnant
with twins. If you've spent your life worrying about your
weight—and most of us have!—it can be hard to let that go.
But take heart. You can lose any excess weight *after* the pregnancy, especially if you breast-feed, which burns off 600 kcal
per day. Meanwhile, work with your doctor to make sure
you're eating enough—especially if you started your pregnancy
at a low weight. (For more on nutrition and weight, see Chapter 7.)

- **Congenital anomalies.** We don't yet understand the relationship, but anomalies in the fetus—known as *congenital* ("from
birth") anomalies—are associated with a higher risk of preterm
labor. Such anomalies are more common in multiple pregnancies, whether they affect one or more fetuses. That's why you
may want to consider amniocentesis and other types of prenatal
tests—they can help you and your doctor evaluate your risk of
preterm labor. (See Chapter 6 for more on testing.)

- **Chromosomal anomalies.** A chromosomal anomaly refers to a
fetus having the wrong number of chromosomes. Down's syndrome is the most common chromosomal anomaly, though there
are others. Many chromosomal anomalies are associated with
structural problems in the fetus, problems that in turn may be associated with preterm labor. These anomalies also seem to be associated with IUGR. You and your doctor should consider
prenatal testing to help evaluate whether chromosomal anomalies are a risk factor for you. (See Chapters 2 and 6.)

- **Fibroids.** Fibroids—benign (noncancerous) tumors in the
uterus—are highly common among women over the age of 40.
Some 20 percent of all U.S. women are affected, and rates among
African-American women seem to be increasing. Normally,

fibroids cause few if any problems to the nonpregnant women who have them, and—in women who are not pregnant—fibroids are relatively easy to remove. However, the hormones stimulating pregnancy may cause fibroids to grow or degenerate (outgrow their blood supply). And this condition can, in turn, cause pain, contractions, or preterm labor. There's some controversy over whether this common condition needs to be treated before pregnancy. Usually, in my opinion, it doesn't—but fibroids do need to be closely monitored.

Another type of problem can occur if two fetuses are sharing space in the uterus with a fibroid tumor: The fetuses may not be getting enough blood, and their growth might be restricted. If you have become pregnant while fibroids are in your uterus, your doctor will want to monitor you closely.

- **Exposure to ionizing radiation (X rays), anesthetic gases, lead.** These toxic conditions can cause congenital anomalies, which, as we've seen, can lead to preterm labor. Of course, you probably don't need to be told to avoid X rays, anesthesia, or lead paint while pregnant! But if you're exposed to any of these substances accidentally, tell your doctor.

- **Auto or bus accident, or other injury.** I surely don't have to tell you to stay out of accidents! But accidents happen, and if they happen while you're pregnant, they are a risk factor for premature labor. A physical trauma to the mother can lead to placental abruption, which can in turn cause contractions to begin. If you're in an accident of any kind, let your doctor know right away. (For more on placental abruption, see the section on "Additional Risk Factors," page 215.) Meanwhile, buckle up! (For more on the proper way to wear a seat belt when carrying a multiple pregnancy, see Chapter 10.)

- **Two or more second-trimester abortions.** Late-term abortions or multiple D&Cs can traumatize the cervix, leading to cervical incompetence—a condition in which the cervix isn't strong enough to carry a baby to term. Be sure you've told your doctor about any history with abortions, so that he or she can monitor the health of your cervix. (For more on cervical incompetence, see the section on "Additional Risk Factors," page 215.)

It can be overwhelming to read through a long list of risk factors, wondering how many of them apply to you. But if you can, try to take it in stride. Paradoxically, knowing about your risk can actually help you to become more relaxed about your pregnancy. Work with your doctor, your birth coach, and your support system to respond to your condition, developing a relaxed but prepared state of mind.

"In some ways, being pregnant with triplets felt like this huge psychological preparation for actually *having* three babies to take care of," Sarah says thoughtfully. "The pregnancy itself felt like such a lot of work and such a lot of risk. But I realized, about one month in, that if I spent the entire pregnancy worrying about what *might* go wrong, I'd miss all the joy of the experience. And if I spent my babies' entire childhood worrying about what might go wrong, I'd miss that joy too. I simply had to decide: Was I going to be anxious, or was I going to commit to feeling good about my pregnancy? Even though I knew the risks were very real, I decided that I'd rather think positive."

Diabetes

As we saw in Chapter 13, diabetes is a frequent complication of pregnancy. Diabetes may be pregestational (either Type 1, insulin-dependent, or Type 2, non-insulin-dependent), or gestational. For more on this topic in general, look back at Chapter 13. Here, we're just going to talk about how diabetes might affect your risk of preterm labor and premature birth.

CHRONIC DIABETES. If you have chronic diabetes, you may already know that the condition increases your chances of having babies with structural anomalies, such as heart disease, forms of spina bifida, and the like. Your babies may also have a tendency to be underweight. Diabetes can cause vascular complications, which in turn can damage the small blood vessels of the kidneys, eyes, heart, and even the placenta. If you do indeed have poor *placental perfusion*—a poor supply of blood to the placenta—your babies may be undernourished and their growth may be restricted.

Again, this is a problem that's even more serious with twins and other multiples, who are already prone to low birth weight. Moreover, if you're diabetic, you need to be monitored for placental insufficiency later in the pregnancy, to make sure your babies are being properly nourished. Finally, you might be prone to *ketoacidosis,* an imbalance of acids and bases in the blood, which can cause problems for your fetuses. Your doctor will be watching for this condition.

For all these reasons, even the diabetic mothers of singletons are often delivered before term, depending on how severe their condition is. The diabetic mothers of twins and other multiples are even more likely to have difficulty with prematurity.

The good news is that it's perfectly possible for you to have healthy babies, even if you do deliver somewhat early. Being monitored closely may take time and effort, but the rewards are well worth it.

My patient Elena had chronic diabetes when she became pregnant at age 32. Her diabetes was not well-controlled, and I was worried that the pregnancy would be filled with complications for her and her babies.

It turned out that I didn't need to worry at all. From the moment Elena saw her twin daughters waving to her from the sonogram screen, she turned into a model patient who surprised us all. She monitored her glucose levels four times a day and kept a meticulous, four-color graph to record every reading. She was rigorous about following her diet—and her care paid off. When she delivered two healthy girls at 37 weeks, she considered it a personal triumph—and so did I.

GESTATIONAL DIABETES. As we saw in Chapter 13, the same placental hormones that create the tendency to gestational diabetes also seem to produce fatter babies. And if your babies are gaining too much weight too quickly, or if you've got polyhydramnios (excess amniotic fluid), you may be facing an increased risk of preterm labor. As we've seen, your body goes into labor in response to a complex set of cues. The extra fetal weight of your babies and a "distended" uterus may help signal your body to go into labor too early.

Once again, if you do have gestational diabetes, it's cause for concern—but not for alarm. The extra monitoring you can expect from your doctor will go a long way toward helping to head off any potential problems that might arise.

Additional Risk Factors

Certain conditions in your placenta, uterus, or genital area can also increase your risk of preterm labor:

PLACENTA PREVIA. In this condition, the placenta is attached to the lower half of the uterus, a position in which it covers, partially covers, or just touches the edge of the cervical *os,* the uterus's mouth. In many cases, during the early stages of pregnancy the placenta lies low within the uterus, but in most cases it gradually moves upward.

However, if your placenta is blocking the cervical opening, even partially, you won't be able to deliver vaginally. And if your placenta is touching the os, even a little, it can cause you to bleed or even to hemorrhage.

Since you're carrying a multiple pregnancy, your placenta is likely to be larger than normal. That's because your babies need a larger placental surface to transmit extra nutrients and oxygens. Unfortunately, your larger placenta also puts you at higher risk of placenta previa, since a larger placenta is more likely to extend down into the cervical opening.

If you have scarred uterine walls, you're at even higher risk of placenta previa. You might have gotten scarred uterine walls from previous pregnancies; cesareans; D&Cs after miscarriage or abortion; fibroids; or uterine surgery.

The key symptom of placenta previa is painless bleeding. Indeed, some 2 to 6 percent of women carrying twins have some *antepartum bleeding* (bleeding before delivery), some of which may be associated with placenta previa.

However, you can also have placenta previa without having any symptoms. As with all the other conditions we've discussed, this is something your doctor should be watching for—in this case, with ultrasound. If your sonogram shows full or partial previa in the second trimester, your doctor will check it again as you get close to term, since only a small percentage of cases persist throughout the pregnancy. (For suggestions on how you and your doctor might respond to this condition if it does persist, see Chapter 15.)

PLACENTAL ABRUPTION. Another possible problem is placental

abruption, in which the placenta detaches itself from the wall of the uterus. You're more likely to have this condition if you're an older mother who has already had a few babies. You're also at higher risk if you smoke, take amphetamines, or use cocaine; if you have high blood pressure (whether chronic or induced by the pregnancy); and if you take aspirin late in your pregnancy. Sometimes a short umbilical cord or an accident can cause this condition as well. A history of placental abruption increases by ten times your risk of abruption occurring in later pregnancies.

Naturally, if you have any kind of injury or accident during pregnancy, call your doctor! The doctor will need to test you after the accident and may want to test you again several hours later or over the next two days.

Like placenta previa, placental abruption is often signaled by bleeding, which is sometimes accompanied by a severe, sharp, sudden pain. There are degrees of placental abruption, from mild to severe. Sometimes this condition shows up on ultrasound—but only in about half of all cases. So your doctor will determine whether you've got placental abruption by taking your history, giving you a physical exam, and keeping close watch over any uterine contractions or bleeding. (For more on treatment for placental abruption, see Chapter 15.)

If you do get into an accident, I'd counsel you to stay as calm as possible until you've checked things out with your doctor. It's perfectly possible that an accident won't do any harm whatsoever to your unborn children, even if you have suffered some kind of injury. My patient Lizzie, for example, happened to miscarry after an accident in a martial-arts class led to a broken toe. I was able to reassure her that it was pure coincidence that her miscarriage occurred on the following day and that the particular martial-arts routine she had worked out for her pregnancy was in fact perfectly safe. (She went on to a successful pregnancy soon afterward—with no letup in her martial-arts practice!)

GENITAL INFECTIONS. If you have any type of genital infection, even one so slight that you don't experience any symptoms, it can release a cascade of inflammatory chemicals that can set off preterm labor or rupture the membranes. This premature rupture of the membranes, as we saw earlier, can lead to early delivery. Genital infections associated with prematurity include bacterial vaginosis, mycoplasma, ureaplasma, gonorrhea, chlamydia, and possibly Group B streptococcus (or "Group B strep," for short).

There's a second problem associated with genital infections. Apparently, if your vagina and/or your cervix are host to some types of bacteria and other microorganisms, an infection can spread into your amniotic fluid. We know this—or at least, we suspect it—because evidence of such infection is often found in the amniotic fluid of women who have undergone preterm labor. The biochemical response that these infections set off seems to trigger the early labor, even if the infection is *subclinical*—that is, without a lot of symptoms in the mother.

Sometimes the only way you know about an infection is by being tested. For example, *Listeria monocytogenes* is a rare bacterium that some mothers pick up from soft cheeses or infected deli meats. The bacteria may then infect the amniotic fluid and the fetus, leading to premature labor. (So during your pregnancy, you probably want to avoid soft cheese.)

KIDNEY AND URINARY-TRACT INFECTIONS. If you've got a severe kidney or urinary-tract infection (UTI), it, too, may be associated with preterm labor. One study of pregnant women with UTIs found that many women had no symptoms but nevertheless showed a significantly lower rate of prematurity when treated with antibiotics than did a control group that was not treated. If you have a history of UTIs, you will probably get monthly urine cultures.

UTERINE ANOMALIES. Sometimes a mother's uterus is not up to the job of carrying a pregnancy to term, especially a multiple pregnancy. If your uterus has an unusual shape or structure, it may not be able to stretch enough to carry even a singleton pregnancy to term, let alone to bear the additional stress of a multiple pregnancy. Even a uterus without any structural problems may have difficulty with the extra stretching involved in carrying a second (or third, fourth, or fifth) fetus.

If you've got a uterine problem, it might be congenital (existing from birth) or from some other factor. Some examples of uterine anomalies are the bicornuate uterus, in which the uterus has two "horns"; the septate uterus, in which there is a dividing septum inside the uterus; and the T-shaped uterus.

A uterine anomaly might show up on a physical exam, a sonogram, or a hysterosalpingogram (not done during pregnancy). A history of recurrent miscarriages or previous preterm labor is one indication of uterine anomalies, and if this is your history, your doctor may already have had you tested.

CERVICAL INCOMPETENCE. Sometimes it's not the uterus but the cervix that has trouble carrying a pregnancy—or multiple pregnancy—to term. An incompetent cervix poses a risk of premature labor because it may dilate (open) prematurely. This dilation, known as *passive dilation* (without contractions), exposes the fetal membrane to infection or rupture, which might in turn lead to preterm labor. Approximately 1 to 2 percent of all pregnant women suffer from cervical incompetence, which is estimated to cause some 20 to 25 percent of all second-trimester miscarriages.

As with uterine problems, cervical difficulties might be congenital and/or in response to trauma—a response to abortions, D&Cs, previous pregnancies, a cone biopsy, or some other specific event. Your doctor's surest indication that you have an incompetent cervix is your experience of previous pregnancies. If you've been pregnant before, and if your cervix dilated painlessly in the second trimester, chances are that you're running the same risk in this pregnancy. Other means of diagnosis are less reliable: passing a dilator easily through the cervical opening, a sonogram, or a hysterosalpingogram. Your doctor may want to place a cerclage—a cervical stitch like a purse string—in the first trimester to prevent dilation. (For more on cerclage and other possible responses to an incompetent cervix, see Chapter 15.)

OLIGOHYDRAMNIOS (INSUFFICIENT AMNIOTIC FLUID). As we saw earlier, your multiple fetuses are surrounded by amniotic fluid. But sometimes there's not enough amniotic fluid.

Insufficient amniotic fluid, known as oligohydramnios, may be associated with renal (kidney) problems in one or more fetuses. Because the fetuses are urinating less, there is less amniotic fluid.

The problem might also also be caused by problems in the placenta. If the placenta isn't transmitting enough oxygen and nutrients to the fetuses, the fetal urine output is lower—a decrease often indicated by a low level of amniotic fluid.

Oligohydramnios seems to be associated with both preterm labor and early delivery. Certainly, if you've got this condition, you and your doctor may want to consider performing a C-section or inducing early labor to protect your fetuses from possible danger. Oligohydramnios can also be associated with twin–twin transfusion syndrome. (For more on that syndrome, see Chapter 13.)

POLYHYDRAMNIOS (EXCESS AMNIOTIC FLUID). Too much amniotic fluid can also be a problem. The uterus—already distended under the weight and size of twin fetuses—is further stressed by the additional amniotic fluid it must carry. This can be very uncomfortable for you, and in some cases, to help you breathe, your doctor may remove some of the fluid.

Excess amniotic fluid might also indicate that your fetuses are suffering from congenital anomalies, a viral infection, or diabetes, all of which are associated with earlier delivery. If your doctor discovers that you have polyhydramnios, he or she may want to do other types of prenatal testing to check out this possibility.

Finally, polyhydramnios is also associated with twin–twin transfusion syndrome. While twin–twin transfusion syndrome doesn't cause preterm labor, it does indicate that one of the twins may be in danger, which may in turn lead your doctor to call for induced labor or a C-section.

PREMATURE RUPTURE OF MEMBRANES (PROM). This syndrome occurs in 5 to 15 percent of all twin pregnancies, with the rate going up for triplets and up still more for quads and quints. If you're carrying a multiple pregnancy, your fetal membranes are more vulnerable, and you might be in danger of PROM.

There are many reasons why a multiple pregnancy can lead to more vulnerable fetal membranes. Your cervix may be ripening too early. Or your fetal membranes may simply have been stretched too far, either because of the multiple pregnancy itself or due to polyhydramnios, or infection may have weakened the membrane.

If your fetal membranes do rupture prematurely, the fluid leaks out, leading to the risk of infection, preterm labor, and early delivery.

As you can see, the best way to avoid PROM is for you and your doctor to keep an eye on the other conditions we've discussed.

Screening

Watch out for any signs of an infection that might set off preterm labor. Tell your doctor if you notice any unusual vaginal discharge, especially if it's accompanied by itching or burning. Even if you have no symptoms, your doctor may want to have you screened for one or more of the bacterial infections most often associated with risk for preterm labor: bacterial vaginosis, trichomoniasis, Group B beta streptococcus, or chlamydia.

Dental Work

Periodontal disease—gum problems—is a possible risk factor, because infections can enter your bloodstream through your bleeding gums. So your preconceptional care should probably include some good dental hygiene, and do keep up with your flossing and dentist's visits throughout your pregnancy.

Coping with the Risks

As you've read through this chapter, you may feel I've asked you to do two contradictory things. On the one hand, I've pointed out a host of problems and asked you to be aware of various types of symptoms. On the other hand, I've suggested that you should approach your multiple pregnancy in a relaxed, positive frame of mind.

"It *is* a contradiction," Sarah agrees. "And despite all my good resolutions, it was often a real struggle to think positive. Plus, I didn't want to be a Pollyanna. If I *was* scared, or upset, or depressed about all the risks I was facing, I didn't want to just bury those feelings."

On the other hand, Sarah says, the techniques she learned for coping with fear and anxiety have stood her in good stead throughout her experience of raising three little boys. "There's *always* something that can go wrong," she says. "And with three babies, there are always *three* things that can go wrong. Or maybe *nine* things that can go wrong—sometimes it seems that the problems just multiply! And if I *didn't* keep a sharp eye out for problems—if I didn't notice when one of them has a cough, or an infection, or seems unusually cranky and might be coming down with something—we'd all be in big trouble.

"Still," she adds, "there *is* a way to stay alert without being anxious. I don't always achieve it, and I often feel totally overwhelmed by all the things that can and do go wrong. But when I can take that other attitude—alert but positive—it's amazing how much it helps. Even if something *does* go wrong, I find I have a lot more energy to deal with it. And everyone around me is much, much happier."

15.

Coping with Preterm Labor

There are four key responses to the possibility of preterm labor:

1. trying to prevent it;
2. maintaining early and adequate weight gain, so that if your babies *are* born early, they will be supported by the highest birth weight possible;
3. responding to specific problems and warning signals;
4. trying to interrupt preterm labor once it begins and preventing its occurrence a second time.

Of course, none of these steps comes with a guarantee. You might do everything suggested in this book and still deliver early. Your doctor might take every measure known to modern obstetrics and still not be able to reverse an early labor. As we saw in the previous chapter, the statistics on preterm labor haven't changed all that much since the 1920s, when most women started having access to modern medical care. What *has* changed are the survival rates for newborns: If your babies *are* born early, there's a great deal that your doctor can do to improve their chances for life and health.

Basically, everything you need to know about steps 1 and 2 is in Chapters 7, 8, and 9. There, as you'll recall, we talked about:

- eating right to ensure early, adequate weight gain;
- coping with emotional stress;
- getting adequate rest and time "off your feet";
- possibly modifying your work schedule, home chores, exercise routine, and other elements of your lifestyle, so that you get the rest you need.

This chapter will lay out what you and your doctor can do for steps 3 and 4:

- respond to specific warning signals;
- interrupt preterm labor if it does begin;
- prevent its occurrence in the future.

Bed rest, a cervical cerclage (a purse-string–like stitch in your cervix), and tocolytic (labor-preventing) drugs are all tools that your doctor has at his or her disposal. You, meanwhile, can commit to good prenatal care, to following the guidelines for bed rest if your doctor prescribes it, and to becoming even more aware of your body so that you recognize preterm labor or other complications if they begin.

A word about body awareness: It can make a surprising difference, as can a patient's commitment to her own vision of her health care. I remember one patient, Miranda, whose ideas of "best treatment" actually contradicted those of most of the hospital staff, myself included. I had prescribed hospitalized bed rest for her, but in many cases, patients are allowed to get up to use the bathroom and take a shower.

Miranda, however, had been infertile for many years, after which she'd had two miscarriages. When she got pregnant with twins, she was overjoyed, and she was determined to carry them for as long as she possibly could. When her cervix was three centimeters dilated at 26 weeks—indicating that preterm delivery was extremely likely—

I admitted her to the hospital, where she took to her bed with a vengeance.

Given her history and the extent of her dilation, we all thought Miranda's chances of preventing preterm labor were extremely low. But this was a woman bound and determined to bring her babies to term, and she decided that complete immobility was the solution for her. She insisted upon bedpans and refused to move from her bed, even to bathe. After the second week, the hospital staff started complaining about the odor, but she was adamant. If there was anything she could possibly do to carry these babies full-term, she was going to do it. Through sheer force of will, she somehow managed to extend a very risky pregnancy to 34 weeks, when she delivered two healthy twin boys.

Of course, in most cases, such extreme measures are hardly necessary. Many mothers of twins, myself included, are perfectly able to lead relatively normal lives for most or even all of their pregnancies. Still, I like to remember this patient as an example of how much difference a person's body awareness and commitment can make when it comes to facing the challenges of a multiple pregnancy.

Preparing for Preterm Labor: Heeding the Signals

HOME FETAL MONITORS. In recent years, many patients have been given home fetal monitors, which can help them become aware of the increased uterine activity that signals preterm labor. Although the monitor doesn't prevent preterm labor, it may help detect it, which in turn might enable the doctor to prescribe bed rest or some other preventive treatment.

The monitor is strapped to the woman's abdomen, usually for an hour twice each day, although some doctors advise recording contractions for a full 24-hour cycle. Some experts recommend that women expecting higher-order multiples—triplets, quads, and quints—use the monitor two or more times a day, until they feel that they can notice contractions on their own.

After recording, the monitor is connected to a telephone line to transmit the data to a medical center, much as a computer modem or fax machine sends data. Thus, several hours of data can cross the phone lines in a matter of minutes. A nurse or doctor at the medical center then decides whether the data warrants a hospital or doctor's visit.

Studies on the usefulness of home fetal monitors are somewhat contradictory. In one study of 45 women with twin gestations, women who used the monitors did notice preterm labor earlier than the control group who relied on self-palpation (feeling your own abdomen to find out what your uterus is doing). As a result, women using the monitors were more than twice as likely to be admitted to the hospital as their cervixes began to dilate. Early admission meant that the women could be given *tocolysis*—medication to stop labor—which has a better chance of working when your cervix is less dilated. So only 7 percent of the women using monitors delivered because of "failed tocolysis," as opposed to 44 percent of the women who did not use monitors. (For more on tocolytic drugs, see page 232.)

Another study compared 52 women using monitors, 57 women performing self-palpation, and 160 women who received neither type of support. All three groups were pregnant with twins—and all experienced the same rate of preterm labor. However, 96 percent of the women using monitors went to the hospital early enough for tocolytic drugs to be effective, as opposed to only 67 percent of the women who performed self-palpation and 27 percent of the control group. The women who had used fetal monitors also gave birth to "older" fetuses, had lower rates of neonatal intensive-care admission, and experienced shorter hospital stays.

On the other hand, several studies contradict these findings. In a collaborative study of 1,292 patients, which included 215 multiple pregnancies, some using monitors and some not, no differences were found in the incidence of preterm labor, the degree of cervical dilation at the time of diagnosis, or the number of preterm deliveries. (However, the study might not have been statistically significant for multiple pregnancies.)

Here's one more interesting twist. A famous study compared three groups: women who monitored their uterine activity and whose data were interpreted by a medical staff; women who used the monitor and whose data were *not* interpreted; and women who were not monitored.

Guess which groups had the lowest rate of preterm labor? If you said, "Women who used the monitors," you would have been right—*regardless of whether their data were interpreted or not.* All women using the monitors, though, got daily calls from someone at the hospital—and that seemed to make all the difference. The actual data were less relevant.

There is some question of whether a multiple mom's perception of contractions is less reliable than those of a woman carrying a singleton. And there are no data comparing the outcomes of multiple moms using monitors with those relying on their own body awareness. So if your doctor advocates the use of home fetal monitors, they may be a good choice for you. In my opinion, though, it's usually more useful to develop the best body awareness you can, to be sensitive to the signs of preterm labor—and to have excellent access to medical care!

BED REST. As we saw in Chapter 9, I don't recommend bed rest as a general preventive measure. However, bed rest in response to certain warning signals is quite another matter. Your doctor may recommend bed rest if you've had any signs of:

- preterm labor, which might happen as early as 20 weeks or as late as 35 weeks (we'll discuss how to recognize preterm labor in a minute);
- cervical change, vaginal bleeding, or other signs of early labor;
- preeclampsia—a high–blood–pressure condition that affects nearly 25 percent of all pregnancies and may become a factor as early as 28 weeks or as late as delivery (for more on preeclampsia, see Chapter 13);
- previous pregnancy complications, including premature delivery, incompetent cervix, or a history of preeclampsia.

If your doctor does prescribe bed rest, either at home or in the hospital, it's important for you to take it seriously. *Stay horizontal.* For a busy woman, especially one with young children at home or with a long list of chores that calls to you from all over the house, the temptation to get out of bed is well–nigh irresistible. But fight the temptation and stay in bed. (For more on bed rest, see Chapter 9.)

My ambitious patient Marsha had to stay in bed for two weeks of her twin pregnancy. With her usual zeal, she brought her laptop, modem, and phone into bed with her, as well as hiring an assistant to work with her at home. Most of us can't afford such extensive changes, but there are other ways to work out the demands of bed rest. Jeannette hired a local high-school student to come by every day after school and do whatever fetching and carrying she needed in the three hours before her husband made it home from work. "Just knowing that Chloe was coming at 3:00 P.M. took the strain off the rest of the day," Jeannette reports. "I could enjoy relaxing, watching videos, sleeping, reading, chatting on the phone, knowing that a real live human being would soon be in the house if I needed her."

If you have other children at home, bed rest will require even more creativity as you decide how best to explain and cope with the situation. If you've been sent to the hospital, for example—which may be the only practical way for a mother to *get* extended bed rest!—your older children may understand that "We don't know when Mommy is coming home," whereas this level of uncertainty might be terrifying to a four-year-old. It's important to find comforting ways to give your children the information they need, while at the same time being honest and straightforward so they know they can count on what you say.

If at all possible, try to schedule "play dates" with your children, either at home or in the hospital. Find ways that they can be close to you without a lot of physical exertion on your part: cuddling, storytelling, singing, drawing pictures, maybe even watching a video. Also do what you can to ensure that other adults are spending "special time" with your children, so that the unborn and newly born multiples don't seem to be getting *all* the attention.

CERVICAL CERCLAGE. As we've seen, one of the possible causes of preterm labor is a so-called "incompetent cervix"—that is, a cervix that opens too early in response to the pressure of the growing uterus and fetus. If you have an incompetent cervix—as evidenced by previous pregnancy history, ultrasound, vaginal examination, or other symptoms—your doctor may put in a cervical cerclage, or stitch, to support the cervix, "sewing" the cervix closed as a purse string closes a purse. Usually, this procedure is done at the end of the first trimester.

A cerclage is a surgical procedure performed in a hospital, under regional anesthesia—usually an epidural or spinal. It requires an initial

Tips for Coping with Bed Rest

- **Look on it as an opportunity.** Are there books you've wanted to read, crafts you've been meaning to resume or take up, videos you've always wanted to watch? Can this be a time for catching up with friends, either by having them visit or by chatting with them on the phone?
- **Give yourself a break.** For many of us, the very idea of "lolling around in bed all day" sounds like a sinful indulgence. But maybe a little R&R is just what your body and psyche need—heaven knows, you probably won't get another chance for several more years!
- **Focus on yourself.** Keep a journal, dream about the future, sort through photographs, reread old letters, or find other ways to reconnect to yourself, your history, your hopes and dreams. Again, you'll soon have two or three eager children to care for, so this time of reconnecting to "just you" might be a valuable opportunity.
- **Reach out.** This is one of those times to let friends, family, colleagues, neighbors pitch in and help. Who wants to take a child-care shift, bake a casserole, drop work off from the office, sign up for a regular phone date so you have something to get you through those long hours of the afternoon? Asking for what you want, and letting people know how much you need them, can really pay off at times like these.

12 hours of complete bed rest after the procedure, then you're usually allowed to get up and go to the bathroom. Some 12 hours later, if no complications ensue, you can continue all normal activities, although sexual intercourse may be restricted for the rest of the pregnancy.

If you have a cervical cerclage, your doctor will probably want to monitor you fairly frequently until delivery. The sutures may be removed a few weeks before your due date or not until labor begins, depending on your doctor's judgment and the type of sutures. If you suffer from infection, bleeding, or premature rupture of the membranes, however, your doctor will need to remove the stitches right away.

As with bed rest, a cerclage is useful in certain circumstances, specifically in response to an incompetent cervix. And, like bed rest, a cerclage is *not* useful as a general prophylactic or preventive measure, even with multiples.

One last word of caution: If you do have a cerclage, watch for the following symptoms. Call your doctor right away and then go straight to the emergency room if you experience:

- pressure in the lower abdomen;
- excessive vaginal discharge;
- vaginal bleeding;
- unusually frequent urination;
- the sense of a lump in the vagina.

Recognizing Preterm Labor

If you do experience preterm labor, it's important to recognize it and respond right away. The technical definition of preterm labor is *cervical effacement and dilation* (the enlarging and opening of the cervix). Here's what you might notice:

- Your pelvis feels full.
- You feel repeated contractions or rhythmic tightening.
- You have an unusual amount of vaginal discharge.
- You're bleeding.
- A rush or trickle of fluid from your vagina signals a ruptured membrane.
- You've got cramps and/or lower back pain.
- You have a general sense that something is "not right."

Remember: Just because you're experiencing these symptoms does not mean that you're going to give birth. There are lots of ways that preterm labor can be interrupted.

Responding to Preterm Labor

Obviously, you'll want to discuss the entire question of preterm labor with your doctor early in your pregnancy. Make sure you understand the signs and symptoms, and go over the procedure your doctor wants you to follow. I tell my patients to call anytime, day or night, if they think they're in early labor, and your physician should have a similar arrangement for you. You should also have a full discussion with your doctor about tocolytic drugs and any other procedures he or she may be planning to follow if you *are* admitted with premature labor.

If you do go into early labor, here's what happens next:

- You'll get a physical exam to evaluate your general health, including a urine sample to check for a urinary-tract infection; a blood-pressure reading; and a measurement of your temperature.
- Your blood count and blood chemistry may be checked.
- Someone will monitor and evaluate your contractions.
- The fetal heartbeats will be monitored. You'll also get an ultrasound, so your doctor can find out how the fetuses are doing, check their weight and position, and examine their biophysical status.
- An EKG may be done.
- Cultures will be taken of your vagina, cervix, and rectum to find out if you've got Group B strep or other infections, which could put your babies at risk during a vaginal delivery. (For more on Group B strep, see Chapter 12.) While the medical staff is waiting for the results to come back from the lab, you'll be given antibiotics, just in case.
- Your cervix will be checked (if there is no leakage of amniotic fluid) manually and possibly by ultrasound.

My patient Karen was admitted to the hospital with signs of preterm labor at 32 weeks. We hydrated her and her contractions gradually subsided, but she had a mild case of pregnancy-induced hypertension, so I thought it best to keep her in the hospital for another week, just in case. "That week was a real test of my faith," Karen says simply. "I had honestly never thought that *anything* could possibly go wrong. Suddenly, I realized that it could."

Other Tests

In some cases of premature labor, especially if the woman's membranes have ruptured, amniotic fluid can be collected from the vagina and sent for evaluation to determine fetal lung maturity. Knowing the level of development of the babies' lungs will help the doctor better determine just how risky a premature birth might be.

Sometimes, amniocentesis is done to discover whether there's any infection. If there is, the doctor may decide that the babies are actually better off out of the womb, and he or she will proceed with a vaginal delivery or a C-section. Amniotic fluid collected from the vagina will also be tested for a bacterial count and culture.

As we saw in Chapter 14, testing the levels of fetal fibronectin and salivary estriol may also tell us whether the uterine contractions that have brought a woman into the hospital actually mean that delivery is imminent. The clinical usefulness of these tests is still being studied, but they are rapidly joining the resources we have to draw on for screening high-risk pregnancies.

- Once your doctor is sure you're all right and has addressed any underlying medical problems, you'll be given fluids, probably intravenously. That's because women who are dehydrated have far more contractions and are at greater risk of preterm labor.
- As you get fluids, your medical team will watch to see how your contraction pattern responds. Possibly, contractions will stop, and you'll be sent home. In some cases, your doctor may still want to admit you to the hospital. If you do go home, your doctor may prescribe bed rest, a cerclage, or both.
- If fluids don't help—or don't help enough—your doctor may respond with tocolytic drugs (see page 232).
- Basically, the less your cervix is dilated when you begin receiving care, the greater your chances of interrupting preterm labor and preventing premature birth:
  - If your cervix is three centimeters dilated, you've got a 20 percent chance of delaying delivery for 48 hours—no matter what age your fetuses are.
  - If you're treated easily in less than 24 hours, you've got more than a 50 percent chance of delaying labor for up to several weeks.
  - If your membranes have ruptured early in the pregnancy, you have a 90 percent chance of delivering that week.

Tocolytic Drugs, Steroids, and Other Medications

Let's go back a step. Suppose your doctor decides to administer medication to try to stop your early labor. What kinds of treatments might you expect?

- **Magnesium sulfate** relaxes the uterine muscle, helping to reduce contractions. It also interrupts the transmission of nerve impulses to the muscles in the uterus. It's administered intravenously and is considered to be safe during pregnancy. It may cause you to feel tired, limp, and probably flushed and overheated as well. If your babies are born soon after you take this medication, their muscle tone may also be decreased.

- **Ritodrine and terbutaline** (Brethine) are also used. In fact, ritodrine hydrochloride is the only drug that is FDA-approved to decrease uterine contractions. These drugs' side effects include a jittery feeling and, in some cases, nausea and headache. Patients with heart problems should not be given these drugs, but other women can safely take them for up to several weeks, although they will continue to feel fidgety and anxious. Often these drugs are given via a subcutaneous pump, which can be used at home.

- **Indomethacin** (Indocin) inhibits prostaglandins, which, as we saw in the last chapter, help stimulate labor. Indomethacin can be given orally or rectally. One of its side effects is to temporarily close the ductus arteriosus—the vessel that allows blood circulation in the fetus—especially if it's given shortly before delivery, so this drug is never given for prolonged periods. (As soon as the medication is stopped, the vessel opens again.)

- **Betamethasone,** a steroid, should always be given to a woman who seems liable to deliver early. The medication helps the babies' lungs to mature faster by stimulating them to produce surfactant, a key chemical needed for the lungs to function after birth. Thus, the drug can increase dramatically the chances of your babies' survival if they are born early—between 24 and 34 weeks. This medication used to be given weekly as two shots, but evidence is now accumulating to suggest that one weekly course may be enough. This is still a controversial area, though, so talk to your doctor to find out more.

- **Nifedipine** is a calcium channel blocker that is as effective as magnesium. However, it might decrease the flow of blood between the uterus and the placenta.
- **Potassium channel openers and oxytocin receptor antagonists** are some of the newer drugs on the horizon.

"I was terrified when I felt those early contractions," Natalie admits. "I was sure I'd be giving birth to two tiny, sickly infants—and I couldn't bear the thought that anything might happen to either one of them. All I could think was, 'Just let me keep them inside for two more weeks.' " In Natalie's case, we were able to stop the contractions with a combination of hydration and magnesium sulfate. "I'm sure that visualization helped too," she insists. "I just kept seeing them safe and protected inside of me—and eventually the contractions stopped."

How Effective Is Tocolysis?

As with bed rest, cerclage, and all the other responses to preterm labor we've discussed in this chapter, none of these medications is useful in *preventing* preterm labor. Tocolytic medication is a useful response to an existing problem, not a general prophylactic measure.

In fact, there's a great deal of controversy over whether tocolysis is at all effective. As with many other aspects of multiple pregnancy, most doctors have anecdotal information that is not necessarily supported by the contradictory studies that abound. It's also true that tocolysis might be effective even if it only holds off delivery for 48 hours, since that's a window of opportunity for giving the fetuses steroids to help mature their lungs and vastly increase their chances of healthy survival.

There's a movement away from the use of two agents at once, especially in the case of twins, as these medications can produce serious side effects in the mother, such as pulmonary edema (water in the lungs).

There's also been no evidence showing that tocolysis is effective for more than 48 hours in the treatment of PROM (premature rupture of the fetal membranes). However, even gaining an extra 48 hours can sometimes enable us to help the babies' lungs to mature and thereby improve outcomes.

After Preterm Labor Has Been Stopped

There's a lot of controversy over what kind of maintenance therapy should be given after an acute episode of preterm labor is over. Some kinds of medications are often administered either orally or subcutaneously. Recent studies of accumulated data showed no improvement in perinatal outcomes and no reduction in incidences of recurrent preterm labor or delivery, so maintenance therapy may not be necessary after all.

16.

Labor and Delivery:
Getting Ready

As your pregnancy progresses, your thoughts may turn from simply making it through the pregnancy to what the actual delivery will be like. In this chapter, I'll help you prepare by letting you in on some of the decisions you and your doctor will be making, both as the delivery approaches and during labor itself. Ideally, you and your doctor will discuss these decisions extensively well ahead of time, so that if complications occur and your doctor has to act quickly, your doctor will be aware of your preferences—and you will understand the decisions that he or she is making. In the following chapter, we'll look at the delivery process itself, from your very first labor pains to the moment your babies emerge.

Like every other leg of your multiple-pregnancy journey, this part of the trip is likely to be full of surprises. But, as with the rest of your pregnancy, it helps to be prepared! The more you know about what to expect, the more easily you'll be able to ride out the changes.

Anticipating Your Due Date

As a woman carrying multiples, you've probably found lots of ways in which your pregnancy differed from those of singleton moms. One of the most important differences involves your due date. While the ideal length of a singleton pregnancy is 40 weeks, the optimum for twins, triplets, and quads is not as easy to determine.

Let's start, not with optimums, but with averages. In the United States, the average term for twins is 36.3 weeks, while triplets average 33 weeks in the womb, and quads are carried for an average of 31 weeks. However, these averages can be misleading, because they conceal the numbers of extremely premature births, which tend to be those with most complications and the most difficult outcomes. For example, 10 percent of all triplets are born before 28 weeks—an extremely high-risk situation.

If you go into labor before 36 weeks, that's considered preterm labor—which is covered in Chapters 14 and 15. But if you've made it to 36 weeks, you and your doctor can pause to congratulate yourselves. You made it! You're now carrying fully developed, full-term babies, which for multiple moms is a real achievement.

How Long Is Too Long?: Deciding Whether to Induce Labor

Over the last few years, we've seen lots of controversy over the optimal time for a mother to carry a multiple birth. At this point, in most cases, if the mother and babies are doing well, most doctors would try to prolong pregnancy to 38 weeks—and would almost certainly induce labor after 40 weeks.

However, lots of factors could influence that decision:

- **How is the mother's health?** A mother with pregnancy-induced hypertension, a diabetes-related complication, or some other health problem may do better delivering earlier—say, at 36 weeks—rather than risking a longer term.
- **How great is the mother's discomfort?** It's a lot of work carrying around even one baby—and when you're carrying two or more, the extra weight and pregnancy-related discomfort seem to increase exponentially. Some women, for example, experience PUPP, a kind of rash that causes them to itch all over. Other women are so large that they have trouble finding a comfortable position for sleeping. Again, all other things being equal, I'd try

to convince a patient to make it to Week 36—but by Week 38, if the babies' lungs are mature and they are of good size, I might consider delivering her. Natalie, for example, was barely sleeping by the time she neared the end of her ninth month.

- **How are the babies doing?** If sonograms and nonstress tests reveal that the fetuses are continuing to grow and develop, there are obvious advantages to keeping the babies "inside" a while longer. However, as pregnancy continues, the placenta does not always provide sufficient nourishment and oxygen to the fetus, especially when it has more than one baby to provide for. This condition, known as placental insufficiency, can restrict the growth of one or both babies (a condition known as intrauterine growth restriction, or IUGR). If a nonstress test reveals that the babies are not active, or if a sonogram reveals signs of IUGR, then I'd probably either induce labor or schedule a cesarean. This was the case with Natalie, whose babies seemed to stop growing by Week 36. "I'd never even considered the possibility of a C-section," Natalie recalls. "I'd always been sure I'd deliver naturally—I didn't even plan on using drugs. But when you told me my babies weren't doing well, Dr. Leiter, I realized that their health was more important than my idea of the perfect birth."

As you can see, it's a judgment call. So from 36 weeks onward, your doctor will probably monitor you and your babies even more carefully than before. That way, if a situation calling for induction or a C-section does arise, he or she will be ready to move.

"I wish these babies were here!": Dealing with the Discomfort

One of the hardest parts of my work as an ob/gyn is when a multiple mom waddles in at 36 weeks, weary of carrying around an extra fifty pounds, exhausted from the demands of a multiple pregnancy, frustrated with her limitations in dealing with job, spouse, other children. "I've had it!" she says. "Induce me!"

Ironically, though multiple fetuses run more risks of placental insufficiency and IUGR, the multiple mom's overdistended uterus also makes labor more difficult to induce. And, as we've seen, there are often medical reasons to try to prolong the pregnancy.

In cases like these, if the babies are in good condition, I'd probably try to convince the 36-week-pregnant mother to tough it out. By 38 weeks, however, if the mother's cervix is ripe and if her babies are in the optimal birth position (vertex/vertex, or both facing headfirst), I'd consider it all right to induce, especially if the mother wished it strongly.

Likewise, if at 36 weeks the mother's blood pressure is up, or if the results of the nonstress tests are not good, I'd consider it important to induce. For example, over the course of her pregnancy, Rosario developed mild pregnancy-induced hypertension (see Chapter 13). By the time she had made it to 37 weeks, her blood pressure was 140 over 90 and she had a low platelet count (not enough red blood cells for her newly expanded volume of blood). I felt strongly that we should stabilize her and deliver as soon as possible.

By this point in her pregnancy, Rosario was exhausted from the extra weight she was carrying and she had also developed PUPP, the rash I spoke of earlier. She was more than happy to have me induce labor.

Natalie, on the other hand, agreed to the C-section I recommended in response to her babies' restricted growth—but she was never really content with the decision. "Even now," she says, "I keep thinking that it was somehow my fault, that if somehow I'd been a better mom, my babies would have been able to keep growing inside me. I know that's irrational—but it's how I feel."

Whenever these decisions have to be made, I remember that obstetrics is an art as well as a science, requiring instinct and judgment as well as medical expertise. This is also when I remember that the pregnant mother and I are very much partners, who need to work together to choose the best course for mother and babies.

How Induction Works

Inducing labor usually isn't a single action but rather a series of steps, each one of which might or might not result in the onset of labor. That's because labor itself is still a mysterious, complicated process, set off by a cascade of cues, each of which seems to trigger another.

There has been a lot of work done on what exactly triggers the labor process, and there's still a great deal we don't know. What we do know is that through most of gestation, the uterus is a relaxed bag of smooth muscles, held shut by a tightly closed cervix, which in turn is kept firm by collagen. As we saw in Chapter 14, during pregnancy the placenta secretes extra progesterone, a hormone that keeps the uterus firm and the cervix closed.

At the same time, however, the placenta is also secreting estrogen, which has the opposite effect: It makes the uterus more likely to contract. If you think of your pregnancy as a "battle" between estrogen and progesterone, during the early part of your pregnancy the progesterone ideally would "win," keeping your uterus relaxed and your cervix closed. At term, however, your estrogen levels are rising as your progesterone levels fall. Contractions begin when your hormonal balance makes that last definitive shift—so that the forces promoting your smooth, relaxed uterine muscles "lose out" to the forces causing those muscles to contract.

Of course, estrogen doesn't produce this effect all by itself. Higher estrogen levels trigger uterine muscle cells to synthesize *connexin,* a protein that links each muscle cell to its neighbor. This linkage helps all the uterine muscle cells to work together to produce your contractions.

Meanwhile, your elevated estrogen levels are setting off yet another process: They trigger the uterine muscle cells to develop receptors for oxytocin, a hormone produced by the pituitary gland that makes your uterine contractions stronger. Indeed, oxytocin itself can induce labor.

Finally, as your uterine muscles get ready for labor, the estrogen in your body also leads to the manufacture of prostaglandins, a hormone that's involved in the menstrual cycle and other female functions. Before birth, however, these extra prostaglandins are manufactured by the placental membranes that cover the cervix. The prostaglandins in turn induce the cervix to produce enzymes that digest the collagen fibers that have been keeping it firm. From being a tough, hard, closed entity, your cervix ripens, becoming soft and malleable. It begins to dilate and, eventually, to open wide enough to allow your babies' heads to pass through.

What does all this mean for the woman who's waiting eagerly for her doctor to induce labor? It means that there are a number of cues we can use to try to trigger the complicated but well-coordinated process of labor. Sometimes even a single cue can start the labor process rolling.

For example, when I began to induce Rosario's labor, her cervix was "unripe." I began treating her cervix with *misoprostol,* a gel that contains a prostaglandin compound, mimicking the natural action of prostaglandins during labor to ripen the cervix.

Sometimes misoprostol is all it takes, and contractions begin. Of course, the whole process was taking place in the hospital so that Rosario and her twins could be carefully monitored.

Eventually the misoprostol took effect and Rosario's cervix began to dilate and efface—but there were still no contractions. I decided to go on to the next step, performing an *amniotomy*—or rupture of the amnion, the membrane surrounding the fetuses—and administering *Pitocin,* a synthetic form of oxytocin, which, as we saw, inspires uterine contractions and makes them come on with more force and frequency. (Pitocin is also used to move things along during a lengthy or sluggish labor, as we'll see in the next chapter.) Pitocin is administered through an IV by means of a carefully controlled pump, which ensures that the chemical is given very gradually, according to the number of contractions and their presumed strength. As it happened, Rosario was very responsive to the Pitocin, and her contractions began almost immediately. Six hours later, she was the proud mother of six-pound twins, a boy and a girl.

Within the Womb: Possible Presentations

One of the main factors that helps me decide how to handle a delivery is what we call *presentation*—the way the twins (or other multiples) are positioned within the womb. The twins' position helps determine whether or not vaginal delivery is possible.

There are five possible presentations (see Figure 1):

- **Vertex/vertex—when both twins present headfirst.** This, of course, is the safest position for labor. All other things being

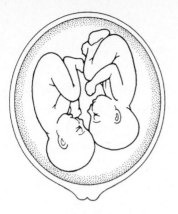

Vertex/vertex

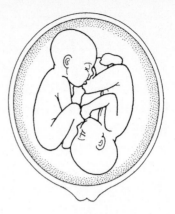

Vertex/breech

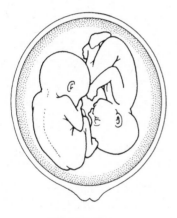

Breech/vertex

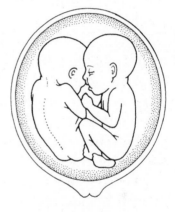

Breech/breech

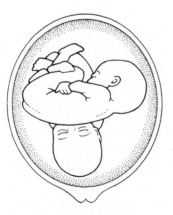

Vertex/transverse

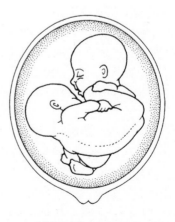

Breech/transverse

Figure 1

equal, I'd advise the mother to opt for vaginal delivery in this case.

- **Vertex/breech—when Twin A presents headfirst, but Twin B presents feetfirst or "tush" first.** Although some ob/gyns immediately call for a C-section whenever a breech is involved, my own practice is to deliver Baby A vaginally and then to try to deliver Baby B as a breech. Of course, I wouldn't attempt this if Baby B is suffering from any kind of distress, if he or she weighs less than 1,500 grams (3⅓ pounds), or if he or she weighs over 20 percent more than the first twin—it's too easy for the bigger baby's head to get stuck. If Baby B seems to be active, healthy, and good-sized, however, I would, with the mother's permission, use the guidance of a sonogram to push Twin B's head down. Alternatively, if it's a footling (feetfirst) breech, I might simply grab the baby's little feet and ease it out. Only a doctor with lots of experience delivering twins and/or breech births should attempt either of these maneuvers, of course; if the doctor isn't comfortable with the procedure, he or she would want to do a C-section to deliver the second baby.
- **Breech/vertex.** In the United States, even a doctor who's comfortable with breech delivery would call for a C-section in this case: There's just too much risk that a breech/vertex configuration could end in interlocking babies, who will not descend properly.
- **Breech/breech.** Some doctors perform a C-section on *every* breech. I deliver breeches vaginally, but, along with a majority of obstetricians, I would call for a C-section rather than deliver two breeches. There are just too many chances for something to go wrong, endangering the two babies and possibly the mother as well.
- **Vertex or breech/transverse lie.** A transverse lie is when the baby is positioned horizontally, with its tush positioned to come out first. Most obstetricians, myself included, would manage this presentation according to the first baby, calling for a C-section if Baby A is breech but trying for a vaginal delivery if Baby A is vertex. If the first baby is delivered vaginally, I might use an ex-

ternal cephalic version to guide the second baby's head down into the birth canal, or I might simply perform a breech delivery.

There is one other situation that calls for a C-section: when your babies are sharing an amniotic sac. (For more on monoamniotic twins, see Chapter 3.) In this situation, it's a lot more likely for one or both of the babies to become entangled in the umbilical cord. The loss rate is so high in this case that virtually all responsible doctors would avoid vaginal delivery.

The Whys and Why-Nots of C-Sections

As Natalie discovered, one of the biggest decisions in multiple pregnancies is whether to deliver vaginally or opt for a C-section. Although sometimes a C-section seems like a miracle of modern science, saving the lives of women and children who in an earlier era would have been lost, we've also seen a vigorous debate among both mothers and doctors over whether the rate of cesareans is too high.

This debate has changed as medical practices have. When cesareans were first performed, they were a far more dangerous business than they are today. Early cesareans required general anesthetic—always a risk—and they posed a fairly high possibility of infection.

Now, however, the procedure is far safer. It's usually done with a less risky local anesthetic. And we now know a lot more about how to prevent and treat infection.

But as cesareans became safer, there was a tendency to resort to them quite often. Both women and doctors may have been tempted by what seemed like a more controllable and more secure option that allowed the mother to bypass the pain, blood, and general messiness of labor. Why shouldn't the busy mother "schedule" her C-section rather than wait upon nature's whims, especially if she has to arrange for work leave, child care, and possible visits from in-laws to help run the household while she is in the hospital? Why shouldn't the doctor avoid last-minute midnight calls while ensuring that he or she will be the one to deliver the babies, rather than relying on whichever doctor happens to be on call that night?

My patient Shirla, for example, came to me at age 37, when she was finally pregnant with twins after 10 years of expensive and often heartbreaking fertility procedures. When her twins made it to 36 weeks, she was sure she was home free. Unlike Natalie, who viewed her cesarean as a defeat, Shirla saw the possibility of a C-section as a safety factor. Why should she risk her precious children in a possibly complicated double delivery? she wanted to know. Wouldn't she be better off scheduling a C-section and delivering her babies in a situation where I would have full control?

As you can imagine, many doctors would agree. These are the attitudes that have led to a sharp rise in C-section rates—which has in turn led many childbirth experts to look for ways to avoid C-sections.

The more I'm called upon to weigh the pros and cons of C-sections, the more complicated I think the issue is. But all other things being equal, I'd prefer my patients to deliver vaginally—even Shirla. Here's why:

1. When vaginal delivery is possible, C-sections don't lead to any kind of improved outcomes for the babies. All the studies agree that C-sections are helpful *only* when vaginal delivery is *not* possible. The single biggest factor in having healthy twins, as we've already seen, is how long they're in the womb. Prematurity, not vaginal birth, is the risk we're most concerned about. Actually, unless there's a specific factor to the contrary, such as a breech presentation, even preterm babies usually do well with vaginal delivery.

2. Vaginal delivery is better for the mother, since C-sections always pose the risks of infection, excessive bleeding, and complications that accompany any operation. If the C-section involves general anesthesia, there's an additional risk and a longer postpartum/postoperative feeling of weakness and exhaustion. Even with a regional anesthetic, it takes longer to recover from a C-section than from a normal vaginal delivery, and the slowly recovering mother now has *two* babies to take care of. And if there *is* some complication that puts one or both twins into the NICU (neonatal intensive-care unit), it's much better if the mother who visits and—hopefully—breast-feeds them there isn't herself recovering from surgery.

3. Uncomplicated vaginal delivery is better for the babies too. Statistics show that there's a slightly higher rate of respiratory distress among babies delivered by C-section. That's because when the baby is delivered vaginally, its head comes out first, while its chest and abdomen are still being squeezed by the uterus. This compression helps force fluid out of the baby's lungs, so that the newborn's first breath doesn't suck fluid into the lungs' tiny air sacs. Some babies delivered by C-section may even experience mild breathing problems, known as TTN—*transient tachypnea of the newborn*—which refers to the fluid retained in the lungs because this chest compression did *not* take place. Most babies recover from TTN within 24 hours, although some may need to be helped along with a little oxygen, or even—rarely—some time on a respirator.

There is one group of babies whose outcomes *might* be improved by a C-section: breech babies weighing less than 1,500 grams (3⅓ pounds). The data on what twins should weigh to warrant a C-section, based on figures for singletons, is suggestive but not conclusive.

When do I schedule C-sections ahead of time? I advise a C-section if:

- there is a placenta previa;
- the mother has any condition that makes vaginal delivery unsafe: for example, uncontrolled pregnancy-induced hypertension or herpes;
- either baby has any condition that makes vaginal delivery unsafe, such as hydrocephalus (enlarged head, which might have difficulty passing through the cervix) or an abdominal wall defect, which leaves part of the bowel exposed;
- Twin A (the twin that will emerge first) is positioned in such a way that vaginal delivery is unwise, such as in a breech (feetfirst) or transverse lie (bottom first);
- in some cases, if the mother has had previous C-sections (see page 246);
- either fetus displays signs of fetal distress or an unreassuring fetal status (as Natalie's babies did).

If You've Already Had a C-Section . . .

Most birthing centers and hospitals will now allow a VBAC—vaginal birth after a cesarean—even for a multiple mom, if all the above conditions for a vaginal birth are met and if the previous uterine incision was made horizontally rather than vertically. (The technical term is an LFT, or *low flap transverse* incision.) The low transverse incision is used far more often these days, as it's a stronger cut and heals better, in addition to being less likely to rupture during a subsequent vaginal delivery. The old "classical" vertical incision makes for an unsafe VBAC, since there is a higher rate of uterine rupture.

If you are having a VBAC, your doctor will make sure that there's a strong multidisciplinary team to support the process: Besides your own ob/gyn, there will be a nurse, a neonatologist (specialist in newborns), pediatrician, and anesthesiologist on hand. You'll be fitted with an IV, and your babies will be monitored via ultrasound and an electrofetal monitor. You'll get an epidural, and your ob/gyn will almost certainly want to perform the delivery in the operating room, so that if an emergency C-section *is* necessary, everything will be in place. There's a 1 to 2 percent chance of a uterine rupture with a VBAC with a singleton (data aren't available for twins)—but in my opinion, the benefits of a vaginal delivery make this a worthwhile risk if all the other criteria are met. In this case, your doctor may avoid using misoprostol (the gel used to ripen the cervix; see earlier section, this chapter), as it may increase the risk of the uterus rupturing.

Making the Decision

As I've said, I myself would perform a vaginal delivery if both twins are in the vertex (headfirst) position, or if the first twin is vertex and the second is expected to be breech, assuming that both weigh over 1,500 grams (3 pounds). Some ob/gyns, however, insist on C-sections for *any* multiple birth involving a breech, particularly if the mother has ever had a C-section before or if the person delivering the baby isn't comfortable with a vaginal breech delivery.

In the end, this is a decision between you and your doctor. My advice is to make sure you each share your philosophies well before the delivery date—and then be flexible. With twins, every delivery is potentially full of surprises, and each situation is different. Ideally, you'll have chosen a doctor you trust enough to help you make the decision that's right for you and your babies.

Doulas, Midwives, and Other Support Systems

Over the past few years, a new kind of childbirth helper has emerged—a doula. A doula (pronounced DOO-lah) is someone whose job is to help the pregnant and early mother in any way possible. In the last few weeks of pregnancy—or, if you can afford it, even earlier—a doula might help with household chores, do baby-related errands (picking up supplies, arranging for delivery of baby furniture), and take on other kinds of "mother's helper" jobs to ease your workload. If your doctor has prescribed bed rest, a doula may well be a necessity to keep your household running. If you have other children, a doula might do some child care—or take on the housework, freeing you for time with your little ones.

During labor, a doula might be present along with the baby's father, a midwife, a birth coach, and other "support systems." Again, the doula's job is to help provide one-on-one support for the mother, at a time when other people in the delivery room may be more focused on the emerging babies.

Statistics show that women with doulas have a lower rate of C-sections than the national average. Perhaps that's because the woman who hires a doula—someone whose sole function is to give *her* support—is better able to assert her wishes and feels more entitled to insist on being listened to. Certainly the woman whose financial situation allows her to hire a doula is more likely to be better-nourished and to receive better prenatal care than her lower-income sister, which may enable her to deliver vaginally. In any case, if the idea of a doula appeals to you, consider hiring one—or, if you can't afford the extra expense, ask a trusted friend, neighbor, or relative to perform this function before or during delivery.

After delivery, of course, a doula can be extremely helpful in taking care of household chores so that the new mother can concentrate on feeding her hungry multiples. We'll talk more about this kind of support in Chapter 19.

Sarah had never heard of doulas before. When I suggested a doula to help her through the bed rest I had prescribed, her first reaction was skepticism. "Philip and I really value our privacy," she said. "I'm not sure we'd do well with another person in the house." When the two of them realized just what was involved in complete bed rest, however, they decided to give the idea a try. Soon Sarah's doula was not only caring for Sarah during what turned into a *very* long month in bed, but she also helped baby-proof the house. She brought Sarah home catalogs and Polaroid snapshots of baby furniture from local stores, so Sarah could have a voice in furnishing their nursery, even if she couldn't get out of bed to shop. And during the hectic first month after the triplets came, their doula helped cook and clean so that Sarah and Philip could focus on their newborns.

"I still don't know how we managed to come up with the funds to pay her," Sarah told me at her three-month visit. "But it was the best money we ever spent. In the old days, I suppose, my mother or Philip's mother would have played that role. But they live hundreds of miles away—and they have their own lives. Thank heavens someone came up with the idea of a doula—she was kind of an instant extended family."

What about midwives? As we've seen in Chapter 5, most midwives won't take patients pregnant with twins, and none will accept patients who are carrying triplets, quads, or higher-order multiples. If you do have a midwife, you and she will ideally have arranged to deliver in either a hospital or a birthing center that's attached to a hospital, so that emergency support systems are immediately available. Likewise, you and your midwife will have chosen a doctor as backup in case of trouble. There's no reason why the midwife can't remain with you throughout the delivery, providing support and assistance whether the doctor is there or not.

Emergency C-Sections

As I've said, sometimes it's necessary to call for an emergency C-section during labor. The word *emergency* may be misleading. There might indeed be a medical emergency, but it may also simply become apparent that a vaginal delivery just won't work. For a number of reasons, the birth may hit a roadblock and not continue as it should, even if there's no immediate danger to mother or babies. Some reasons for C-sections during labor include:

- **Babies who don't fit.** We may not know whether the babies are too large for the mother's pelvis until the delivery begins. If this becomes apparent, however, I'd call for a C-section, since the babies could eventually go into distress if they can't emerge from the womb.
- **Babies who aren't positioned well or who don't descend properly.** Again, this isn't always apparent until the birthing process begins. It's one of the reasons for monitoring mothers—especially multiple moms—and for examining them carefully when active labor begins.
- **Interlocking twins.** When babies "interlock," their heads are positioned so closely together that they won't descend properly. Alternatively, one baby's feet may be obstructing the other one's head.
- **Fetal distress.** This comes in various degrees of severity, and it's one of the reasons to monitor babies closely, especially in multiple births. If a baby's heart rate suddenly goes down, for example, the baby could become hypoxic (deprived of oxygen), and I'd intervene as quickly as possible. Babies who've suffered IUGR are more likely to experience fetal distress, as are babies whose placenta has become too "tired" to support them properly. Ironically, although we always want to prolong pregnancy to a reasonable term, longer-term babies also face more risks of IUGR and placental insufficiency, which could complicate the birth process.
- **Active herpes virus.** If the mother has herpes that is active on the day she goes into labor, the babies might be exposed to the virus as they pass through the vagina. Since newborns' resistance to infection may be relatively low, many doctors won't want to risk infection.
- **Placenta previa.** A mother with this condition risks excessive bleeding during delivery, endangering herself and her babies. A

C-section offers the doctor a better chance to prevent and control bleeding.

- **Diabetes, preeclampsia, or other maternal conditions.** In some cases, the mother will have a condition that puts her at risk for vaginal delivery. If her high blood pressure has not responded adequately to treatment, for example, it may be safer to deliver her babies by C-section than to allow her to have a vaginal delivery.

Anesthesia

If I do have to perform a C-section, I usually recommend a spinal, in which the anesthesia is injected directly into the cerebrospinal fluid—and the mother remains awake. Spinal anesthesia lasts for about an hour and a half, which is usually more than enough time to complete the procedure.

Another possible anesthetic is an epidural, administered by a catheter, which also numbs the mother only from the waist down. Other medications may also be given through an IV to help with any discomfort during delivery. Afterward, such pain medication as Duramorph (a form of morphine) might be given to the mother through the catheter as well. (See Figure 2.)

When C-sections first became widely used, they involved general anesthesia and were treated like any other operation. Today, they're coming to be viewed as part of the birthing process—which means that the baby's father, and perhaps also the birth coach(es), doula, midwife, and other support systems, might be present. Many couples are committed to having the baby's father (or the mother's partner) hold the newborn as soon as possible, even after a cesarean. ("At least my partner, Janet, got to be with me during the procedure," Natalie says of her cesarean. "And I'm so glad she got to hold the babies so soon! At least they had a chance to bond.")

Sometimes, the mother requires general anesthesia. In some rare cases, such as when the umbilical cord is *prolapsed,* or falls back into the womb, a C-section can't be done with a local anesthetic. If the conditions of a possible C-section are important to you and your

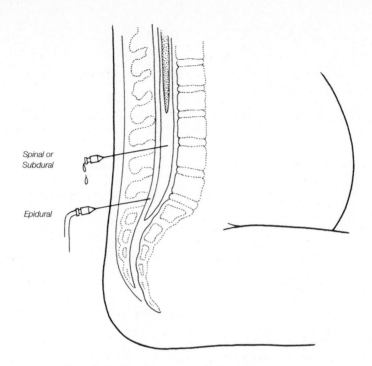

FIGURE 2. With an epidural, the needle does not penetrate
the dura as with a spinal or subdural.

partner, discuss the possibility with your doctor ahead of time and
make whatever arrangements the hospital requires.

C-Sections and Higher-Order Multiples

In the United States, virtually all triplets and higher-order babies are
delivered by C-section—the experience of Phoebe, the character
pregnant with triplets on the sitcom *Friends,* notwithstanding! There
has been some experimenting with vaginal delivery for triplets in Eu-
rope, but almost no hospital will allow this in the U.S.—there are just
too many things that could go wrong by the third baby, and three babies (let alone four!) are just too hard to monitor throughout a long
labor and delivery. Too many things can change too quickly—and it's
too easy for the cords to get entangled.

As we just saw, however, C-sections can be done with regional
anesthesia, allowing you to bond with your babies soon after they

come out and to participate in the birth process at least to some extent. That's what we did with Sarah, whose triplets arrived healthy but somewhat small at 32 weeks. She stayed awake during the entire procedure, and although we needed to make sure each of her triplets was all right, she and Philip were able to hold them soon after the birth.

If You Have a C-Section: What to Expect

If you do have a C-section, here's what happens after anesthesia is assured:

1. First, your abdomen will be swabbed with iodine soap, as a guard against infection.

2. Next, your doctor will make an incision on the lower part of your abdomen. The incision is known as a "bikini cut," since it's supposed to be made in a place that could be covered by a bikini. Usually the cut is horizontal, but if complications are anticipated, the cut may be vertical.

3. After cutting through your skin, fat, and muscle and retracting your bladder, your doctor will proceed to make an incision in your uterus, usually transverse (horizontal), in the lower part of your uterus, so that you could have a vaginal birth in the future.

4. The membranes will be ruptured and the first baby will be lifted out of the uterus. His or her cord will be clamped and cut. If the baby is healthy, he or she can be handed to your partner to begin the bonding process before a pediatrician or nurse takes the baby for testing. If there's any doubt about the baby's health, of course, a doctor or nurse will take the baby right away.

5. Meanwhile, the membrane of the second baby is ruptured and the second baby will be delivered. His or her cord will also be clamped and cut. Again, this baby may be given to your partner, or it may be important for a pediatrician or nurse to take over.

6. Your doctor will deliver the placenta(s), making sure that the uterus is contracting well.

7. Finally, your doctor will sew up the incisions. If you've had a local anesthetic and if there are no medical problems, you'll be able to hold one or both babies soon after that. If you've had a

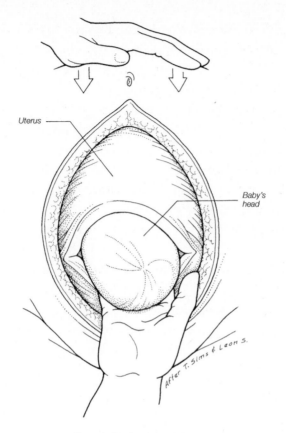

Uterus

Baby's head

After T. Sims & Leon S.

FIGURE 3. Cesarean Birth

general anesthetic, and if the babies are in good shape, you'll be able to hold them as soon as you come out of anesthesia.

Who's in the Delivery Room?

If you do have a C-section, the delivery room is likely to seem quite crowded—especially since you're giving birth to *two* babies. Here's who you can expect to join you in the delivery room:

- **Anesthesiologist**—the person responsible for administering anesthesia; usually sits at the head of the bed.
- **Ob/gyn**—your doctor, who will perform the operation and deliver your babies.

- **Ob/gyn's assistant**—the doctor assisting at the operation.
- **Scrub nurse**—the surgical nurse who hands instruments to the doctor.
- **Two pediatricians**—one for each baby.
- **Neonatologist(s)**—if the babies are premature.
- **Pediatric nurse**—to assist the pediatricians; more than one nurse might be called in if there are complications.
- **Respiratory therapist**—to help the newborns breathe; especially important in case of premature delivery, when the babies' lungs are not yet fully developed.
- **Circulating nurse**—to coordinate the activity and assist in other ways.
- **Medical students, residents, and other learners and helpers**—especially if you're giving birth in a teaching hospital, as most hospitals are; a multiple delivery is both a risky procedure and an opportunity for learning, so be prepared for a variety of learners and helpers to attend the "main team."

17.

Labor and Delivery: What to Expect

Congratulations! You've made it to full term. Now, instead of worrying about extra contractions bringing on premature labor, you just can't wait for that first contraction. You're hoping for a safe delivery of two healthy babies. What can you expect now?

The State of Your Twins

As you reach the end of your term, your twin babies are probably just a bit lighter than the average singleton of the same age: 3,200 grams each (7 pounds), as opposed to the 3,400 grams (7½ pounds) average for singletons. They can be up to 50 centimeters in length. One of their main developmental tasks is storing body fat, which will help them maintain their body temperatures after they are born. Although your doctor will be monitoring you and your twins regularly, ultrasound assessment is not quite as reliable as before, since your babies are bigger and there is less amniotic fluid surrounding them.

Signs of a Change

How do you know that your body is getting ready for labor? Every woman's body is different, of course, but here are a few of the telltale signs that you'll probably notice during the last few weeks of your pregnancy:

- **More Braxton-Hicks contractions.** Many women report feeling contractions for several days preceding their labor. If you get these contractions late in the evening, you might even fall asleep without noticing that they have stopped. The way you can tell true labor, of course, is that the contractions *don't* stop—and if you fall asleep, they'll wake you up! ("I had so many Braxton-Hicks contractions the week before I delivered that I practically didn't notice when the real thing came long," Vanessa recalls. "Then all of a sudden, I was like, 'Hey! This *hurts!*' ")

➤ ALERT: If you notice four or more contractions in a single hour and you are less than 36 weeks pregnant, lie down and drink some fluids. If the contractions persist, or if they are associated with blood or fluids, call your doctor right away.

- **A "full" feeling in the pelvis.** As your babies move into position, you may feel them pressing on your pelvic bone. Some women even feel as though their hips are getting wider.

- **Changes in vaginal discharge.** Often, as women approach their due dates, their vaginal secretions become thicker and more plentiful. This is part of the "mucous plug" that is covering the opening in your cervix.

- **Spotting or bleeding.** As your body prepares for labor, your cervix effaces (becomes thinner) and dilates (opens). As a result, some bloody mucus during this time isn't unusual.

➤ ALERT: If you notice enough blood to fill a menstrual pad, call your doctor right away.

- **Amniotic fluid leaking from your vagina.** This might signal the onset of labor—but you might also notice some fluid while you're still several days away from delivery.

> ALERT: If you notice *any* amniotic fluid, report it to your doctor right away. He or she can decide whether or not it warrants a trip to the hospital.

"It seemed like I was on the phone with you every other day," Zoe recalls. "One day it was mucus, the next day, leaking fluid and some spotting. When the contractions finally started, though, there was no mistaking them. That was the one part of my twin pregnancy that felt *exactly* the same as my previous two!"

Preparing a "Battle Plan"

As you move past your 34th week, your doctor will probably be examining you once a week. You'll get a pelvic exam, and your doctor will also notice how dilated your cervix is—an indication of how close you are to term. He or she will also note the positions of your babies.

What your doctor finds on these final visits helps him or her decide how to respond to your first contractions. If your cervix was not particularly dilated at your last exam, and if it's your first delivery, you can probably expect a longer labor. So unless you're planning a C-section, your doctor will probably want you to stay at home until contractions are coming regularly every 5 or 10 minutes—which might not happen for another 12 to 24 hours.

However, your doctor may see that your labor is proceeding more quickly. Perhaps your cervix is dilated, your babies seem to be in position, and/or you've delivered before. Or you may be facing a potentially slow labor—but your doctor is concerned about some complications. In those cases, you'll probably be told to come to the hospital somewhat sooner, just in case. Likewise, if you're delivering early, if you've had one or more children before, or if you're already dilated, your doctor will want you to come in earlier.

As always, communication is absolutely key. Of course, you always listen carefully to your doctor during office visits—but these last few visits before the babies come are an especially important time. Make sure you understand clearly the doctor's instructions on what signs to notice and when to call. Every case is different, and it's up to your doctor to tell you which signs count as "normal" and which constitute a "special alert" requiring an immediate call.

In any case, you'll want to be prepared. Have your doctor's number handy. Pack your bag ahead of time or have a checklist ready of what to take. Have a sitter or relative standing by to take care of the children you leave at home. Many women go into labor in the middle of the night—to the ob/gyn, it seems like most!—so be sure that any child-care arrangements you make include a "midnight option."

"My mother had dibs on the first two weeks after the babies were born, and Ira's mother was coming for the second two weeks," Miriam recalls. "We had explained to both of them that the babies could come any time, that the timing of a twin pregnancy was especially tricky. One night during my last month, my mother surprised us by just dropping by around dinnertime, which even for her was fairly unusual. Somehow she ended up staying so late that we *had* to put her up—and sure enough, that night I went into labor. She was right there waiting for me when we brought the babies home from the hospital—and she'd even had time to go shopping!"

"We had already decided that Nick's sister, Rosie, would be the child-care person while we were at the hospital," Zoe says. "Sean and Lissa both adore her, and she'd been spending 'quality time' with each of them the whole time I was pregnant. We got her a cell phone, just for the occasion, and she agreed to be on twenty-four-hour standby. And in fact, we did have to call her at three in the morning—and bless her, she came right over."

The First Stage: Latent Labor

The first stage of labor is known as *latent labor.* Here's what you might expect:

- **Contractions.** As you know, a contraction is the movement of your womb compressing, helping to push the babies through the birth canal and out into the world. In this early stage, contractions may last up to 45 seconds. Most women find them painful, but at this stage, some don't. In latent labor, contractions come as far apart as half an hour, or as close together as five minutes. In

What to Take to the Hospital

Of course, you already know about taking sleepwear, a robe, your nursing bras, toiletries, and anything else that might make you comfortable during a stay that might last up to a week or more. Here are some other suggestions that might make labor and recovery more pleasant:

- Light reading—you might want a variety of choices, depending on your energy;
- Walkman, CD player, or boom box, and tapes or CDs—you might want to play music during labor and the birth and to listen quietly to music during your hospital stay;
- Sleep mask;
- Pedialyte, Gatorade, and other nourishing drinks;
- Healthy food and snacks (for a break from hospital food): whole-grain cereal, fresh and dried fruit, nuts, rice cakes, nut butters;
- Photographs, cards, a poster, your children's drawings, or anything else that you like to look at;
- Pleasantly scented oils and lotions.

most cases, you don't need to call your doctor, especially if it's the middle of the night. Just check in when contractions are ten minutes apart—or if you're noticing some of the danger signals I describe below. Of course, in this as in all things, you should get specific instructions from your own doctor before labor begins.

- **Cervical effacement.** When labor begins, your cervix is effacing—getting thinner. Usually, your cervix will dilate—open up—to 2 or 3 centimeters in this phase, compared to the 10 centimeters you'll achieve later on. But if this is your first delivery, your cervix may be only slightly dilated. Don't be discouraged: You'll get there eventually!
- **Babies moving.** Throughout latent labor, your babies will continue to move pretty much as they have been during the last few weeks of your pregnancy.

TRUE VS. FALSE LABOR: HOW CAN YOU TELL?

Feature	False Labor	True Labor at Term
How often contractions come	Irregular, don't come more often	Regular, come closer and closer together
How long contractions last	Irregular	45 to 60 seconds
How intense contractions are	No increase in intensity, not especially uncomfortable	Become more and more painful
If you change your body's position . . .	. . . contractions go away	. . . no change, or contractions increase
Where contraction is located	Lower abdomen	Upper abdomen, or the lower back, radiating to the lower abdomen

➤ ALERT: If you have the sense that your babies have stopped moving, or that they have radically altered their pattern of movement, call your doctor right away.

• **Fluid leaking.** When the fetal membrane ruptures, you'll notice lots of leaking fluid. In popular language, your water has broken! This isn't a danger signal—it's a perfectly normal part of every birth—but you should report it to your doctor, so he or she can best decide when you need to go to the hospital. With multiples, it's usually sooner!

➤ ALERT: If your fluid isn't clear, report that to your doctor right away. You might be seeing traces of *meconium,* a greenish-brown substance indicating that your babies have moved their bowels in utero. Some 10 to 15 percent of all pregnancies are complicated by this condition. If this is your case, your doctor will want to monitor you more closely, for if your babies go into fetal distress while meconium is present, they're at risk for *meconium aspiration syndrome*—a serious condition in which they are literally breathing in their fecal matter. However, meconium is common in deliveries, so don't worry. If there's no fetal distress, and if your doctor makes sure to have the right kind of suctioning at birth, your babies should do just fine.

➤ ALERT: If you find blood in your amniotic fluid, or if you are bleeding heavily, call your doctor right away.

- **Diarrhea.** The days of the routine enema upon arrival at the hospital are long gone, but lots of women do notice diarrhea during the early part of labor. That's an apparent response to prostaglandin, a hormone that, as we've seen, is involved in the onset of labor. Stay hydrated and be patient.

- **Mucous discharge.** At some point, you will expel your mucous plug, which closed the entrance to the cervix. A little blood in the mucus is perfectly normal, so don't be concerned.

➤ ALERT: If you notice heavy bleeding along with the mucus, call your doctor right away.

For couples who are having their first child—especially with a twin pregnancy—it's hard to rest and relax during the latent stage of labor, but honestly, that's the best thing you can do for yourself. You've probably got from 12 to 24 hours of latent labor—followed by one of the most arduous tasks of your life. So pace yourself, and, if you can, pamper yourself a little. Think of yourself as an athlete resting up, physically and mentally, before the big game.

You will want to eat lightly in very early labor, as well as drink lots of fluids. Gatorade, Powerade, soups, broths, and Pedialyte freezer pops are all good sources of needed nutrients (again, think like an athlete!). Stay away from greasy foods—they might make you nauseous, and you're more likely to vomit later in labor—but do eat foods you enjoy and try to give *yourself* a little "babying."

On the other hand, if you know you'll need a cesarean section and you go into labor, call your doctor right away and *don't eat*. A C-section is just like any other kind of operation—best to have it on an empty stomach.

Many couples are quite scrupulous about recording every single contraction during this time, but I personally don't think it's necessary. Far better for you both to get some sleep, if you can, rather than sitting rigidly over the stopwatch, alert for the next event. You'll notice when contractions are coming every ten minutes, especially because by then contractions usually last up to a minute and are quite painful. Most doctors don't need a detailed record of what happens before then.

"Barry went out and rented lots of videos as soon as I went into labor," Shana recalls. "We just sat around watching movies on TV, and I tried to nap as much as possible. Boy, did I appreciate *that* during the next phase of labor!"

The Second Stage: Active Labor

Active labor is the period in which your babies are moving more quickly through the birth canal and your cervix is dilating more rapidly. The first major decision to be made in this stage is the point at which you should come in to the hospital.

Ideally, your own doctor will be on call when you go into active labor. Since your doctor has recently examined you, he or she will have a good sense of how your pregnancy was progressing and how quickly your labor is likely to proceed.

Possibly, though, you'll be delivered by another physician, either a colleague from your doctor's practice or someone on call at the hospital. In our practice, we make every effort to introduce patients to their "backup" doctors well ahead of time—though some patients are just as happy to postpone the meeting until they're actually on the labor floor. If meeting the person who will supervise your delivery is important to you, discuss this with your doctor sometime in your last trimester.

If you do have to call another doctor, he or she will probably ask you several questions to determine exactly when you need to come to the hospital. Try to have answers ready to queries like the following:

- When was your last exam?
- How far dilated were you then?
- How effaced were you?
- Were your babies' heads down? What did your doctor tell you about what position they were in?
- Are your babies moving? What do you notice about their movement?
- Are you bleeding? How much?
- Have you noticed any other discharge? What color is it?
- Has your water broken yet?

Whether you're talking to your own doctor or to a new physician, you'll probably be told to go to the hospital once your contractions become regular, rhythmic, and about ten minutes apart. Ideally, you'll spend at least part of the latent labor stage at home, while spending the active labor stage in the hospital.

At the Hospital

When you get to the hospital, you'll probably be examined fairly soon. A doctor or nurse will check the following signs to see how far along you are:

- How dilated is your cervix?
- How effaced is your cervix?
- How are your babies positioned?
- How far down in your pelvis are they?

You'll also be asked again about how your babies are moving, when your water broke, and anything else you've noticed so far. And you'll be given a sonogram, to determine fetal position and measure your fluid levels.

"When we finally got to the hospital, I felt like I was in one of those awful TV comedies," Shana recalls. "My husband, Barry, was the classic basket case—the nurse asked him about our insurance three times and he just stared at her like she was speaking Greek. I was actually fairly calm and collected, and I answered all the questions that got us admitted. But once you had actually examined me, Dr. Leiter, it finally hit home—I was having a baby! At that point, *I* fell apart and Barry was just a rock. It was like that for most of the first part of labor—we just took turns falling apart."

Monitoring Your Labor

The next step is to begin to monitor your babies. Because twins are considered a high-risk pregnancy and because there are *two* babies to watch out for, your doctor will almost certainly want to keep a closer watch on you and your babies than he or she would on a singleton delivery.

The main device on which your health-care team will depend is the fetal heart monitor. A fetal heart monitor, as the name suggests, monitors the heart rate of the fetus and is used to detect fetal distress during labor.

As with many aspects of birth, fetal heart monitors were once routine and are now controversial—for singleton pregnancies. The controversy centers on whether a birthing woman needs to be hooked up to a monitor rather than simply being monitored at regular intervals. The use of the monitor is seen by some as an unnecessary intervention, preventing the woman's free movement and making a natural process overly medical.

Whatever the pros and cons of fetal monitoring in a singleton pregnancy, most doctors believe that there is *no* justification for not using a fetal heart monitor during a multiple pregnancy—and I agree. Although there's no statistical evidence to show that fetal heart monitors improve outcomes in low-risk situations, I and every ob/gyn I know have plenty of anecdotal evidence in which a fetal heart monitor allowed us to detect a problem in time to intervene.

Where there *is* room for debate is in *how* fetal heart monitors should be used. Because the woman hooked up to a monitor can't walk, squat, or do any of the other physical activity that might ease her pain and speed her labor, ideally, a woman in labor won't be monitored continuously. The American College of Obstetricians and Gynecologists' (ACOG) guidelines recommend that in low-risk singleton births, the mother be monitored for only 5 of every 15 minutes—slightly more often for twins. That way, the mother can walk around between times.

However, there's not always sufficient nursing staff to check in on the mother every 15 minutes and conduct the 5 minutes of monitoring. If the mother is hooked up permanently to the monitor, she doesn't have to be watched as closely. The monitor will simply begin to beep when it registers distress, and the mother or her birth coach can call the nursing staff.

If being able to move freely during labor is important to you, this is yet another issue that you, your doctor, and your support people (partner, birth coach, midwife) should work out with the hospital you've chosen. You don't want to arrive at the hospital in labor only to find yourself arguing about the fetal heart monitor.

Many birthing rooms are equipped with "twin monitors," which can monitor and record two fetal heartbeats at a time. Otherwise, you'll probably be hooked up to two monitors. Obviously, what your doctor is trying to avoid is a situation in which only one baby's heartbeat is heard—twice—while the second baby's heart is never heard at all. If it turns out to be hard to monitor both babies, we might try another strategy once the membranes are ruptured: One baby might be monitored from the outside (through the mother's belly) while the other is monitored from the inside (we'll extend a clip through the mother's vagina to attach to the baby itself). This procedure will also allow the mother a bit more freedom of movement.

In addition to the fetal heartbeat monitor, you'll also be fitted with a belt that keeps track of your uterine contractions. To keep you nourished and hydrated, and for emergency access to medications, you'll also have an IV. Because of the possibility of an emergency C-section, you won't be allowed to eat during active labor, so you'll need an IV to keep your strength up—and to keep you hydrated, if you're having an epidural (otherwise, your blood pressure might drop).

Interventions: Pitocin

Pitocin, as we saw in the previous chapter, is used to induce labor. It's also used when labor fails to progress. If the babies are active and labor is proceeding quickly, Pitocin probably isn't necessary, but I think it's an important tool to have in reserve. A twin labor is especially likely to run into situations where labor isn't progressing, or isn't progressing quickly enough: Your uterine muscles have been stretched so far, they may have difficulty contracting properly, or they may tire more quickly from the effort of contracting. Pitocin can help the uterus work more efficiently, especially in long labors where it's easy for both mother and babies to tire.

"Thank heavens for Pitocin," Miriam says bluntly. "I'd been in labor for about ten hours—remember?—when you told me that you were going to give me something to help the labor along. I know it helped physically, but it helped psychologically too. I thought, 'Okay, I've got help, we've got drugs, everything is fine. Sooner or later, this *will* be over.' "

Anesthesia: Pros and Cons

As with C-sections, the winds of fashion have blown in various directions where anesthesia and natural childbirth are concerned. Some of my patients want to experience every moment of childbirth, unhampered by drugs. Others turn eagerly to the wonders of modern medicine.

I've had some patients ask me whether, as multiple moms, they can expect unusually long and painful labors. Certainly twins and other multiples do tend to have long labors, though not necessarily longer than singletons. On the other hand, multiples tend to be smaller—so they may actually be quicker and less painful to deliver.

As always, I try to be realistic and to encourage my patients to do the same. If a woman is bearing two eight-pound babies and she's only two centimeters dilated, she's going to face a very long, painful labor, and she'll almost certainly need some help to make it through. Even in shorter labors, many women find the pain overwhelming, and they often deal with it by becoming tense and tight. Ironically, this response lengthens the labor and prolongs the pain. A woman who is experiencing less pain may be more relaxed and more able to dilate quickly.

Where twins are concerned it's especially important to consider regional anesthesia, for if the second twin turns out to be a breech, I may need to reach inside and extract it, or I might want to manipulate the mother's abdomen from the outside, a maneuver known as an external cephalic version. (For more on breech births, see page 275.) Without anesthesia, these procedures can be uncomfortable. Also, if a C-section has to be done, having the epidural in place can help us avoid general anesthesia.

This is a time when a solid doctor–patient relationship really pays off. If I can trust my patient to tell me what she's feeling, and if she can trust me to make the decisions that are best for her and her babies, we can get through this difficult time together. It's also a moment when good birthing classes make a huge difference, as the mother and her birth coach(es) draw on all the pain-relief and relaxation techniques that they've learned.

"I'd never needed or wanted anesthesia for my other two births," Zoe says. "But it was absolutely clear to me that this time was different. I don't know if it was having twins, or being ten years older, or just one of those things that make every birth unique. But I could tell that if I didn't get some help this time, I'd be one big tense ball of pain."

Marsha, on the other hand, had plunged into a birthing class on the Bradley method with her usual "all-or-nothing" enthusiasm. She was absolutely committed to doing without anesthesia, a preference of which her doula, her husband/birth coach, and her friend Lydia had all been made aware. I'll never forget the sight of those three people working with my determined patient—the doula rubbing her back, Lydia feeding her ice chips, her husband's eyes fixed on hers as he kept her focused on her breathing and relaxation techniques. When Marsha made it through a 24-hour labor and delivered two six-pound boys "drug-free," we were all somewhat in awe.

Types of Anesthesia

Once you're in active labor—whether spontaneous or induced—you may want to have an epidural. This form of anesthetic numbs the lower half of your body, leaving you awake and conscious.

Epidurals are administered through a catheter inserted into your epidural space, right outside the spinal cord. Once the catheter is in place, the medication can be delivered quite quickly and will take effect in a matter of minutes.

I would encourage patients who are unsure about whether or not they want anesthesia to have the catheter fitted before delivery, so that the epidural is available if they want it. It's fairly easy to adjust the dosage—or not to administer any medication at all. But both my patients and I tend to feel more comfortable knowing that relief is available, particularly if a C-section or manipulation of the babies turns out to be necessary.

Neither a spinal nor an epidural will hurt your babies in any way. You just have to be sure not to lie flat on your back, as your large uterus will press down on your vena cava—a major blood vessel—causing potential problems with circulation. If you're most comfortable on your back, use a pillow as a wedge to elevate one hip.

One disadvantage of an epidural is that you can't walk around during labor, even though many women have found that walking both relieves labor pains and helps move the birth process along. A so-called *walking epidural* leaves you enough sensation to push and participate in your delivery. However, even a walking epidural numbs the lower half of your body. Although theoretically the medication is diluted enough to allow you to move your legs, everyone's response is different. Your doctor probably won't want to take the chance that you're the one woman who reacts more sensitively to a "low" dose, loses all feeling in your legs, and falls to the ground. In any case, the need to monitor both your twins throughout active labor may make it hard for you to move around freely. At least the epidural allows you to feel some of the process, leaving you able to participate in the delivery.

There is a 1 percent risk of headache with an epidural, though the headache can be treated. And, very rarely, there may be some other complications, including bleeding or infection. However, an epidural is a very common procedure, and complications are very rare.

You may also be given painkillers during early labor, such as Demerol (meperidine hydrochloride) or Stadol. If you get these medications, they'll be administered through your IV, and you'll get them fairly early in the labor process. They might make you drowsy, which is fine when you're just having contractions but not so good later on when you need to push. And, unlike epidurals, this type of pain reliever does cross the placenta, making your newborns drowsy as well. Your doctor wants your babies to be born wide awake and breathing at full strength—especially if they're premature—so he or she won't take the chance of giving you pain medication that might depress your babies' respiratory systems. Demerol, Stadol, and other pain relievers last for about 90 minutes, so you won't get them within two hours of your expected time of delivery.

"I was grateful for the pain relief," Zoe recalls of her own experience with Demerol during labor, "but I must admit, I didn't like feeling drowsy. It made me feel more out of control—as though I were cut off from a process that, while painful, was also tremendously exciting."

"I *loved* those painkillers," Shana says. "I actually enjoyed the drowsiness, because it was kind of like a little time-out."

As Your Labor Progresses...

Now that you're in active labor, your cervix will be dilating a bit faster. The average rate for a singleton birth is 1.2 centimeters per hour (if it's a first delivery) or 1.5 centimeters per hour (if the mother has already had one or more children). However, twins are different, and your rate of dilation may be somewhat slower. In any case, you'll probably continue with contractions at one to five minutes apart for the next six or seven hours, until your cervix is about ten centimeters dilated. If your contractions slow down, or if your cervix isn't dilating properly, your doctor may give you Pitocin to help move things along.

When your cervix is fully dilated, your first baby's head should just be descending into the pelvis. At this point, you'll be asked to *push*—to bear down through the uterus and in the pelvic region to help ease the baby through the birth canal and out through your vagina.

Also at this point, your doctor may be considering a C-section. The classic med-school formula is known as the "Three P's": pelvis, passenger(s), and power. Is your pelvis big enough for your babies to pass through easily? Are your little passengers doing well? And is your uterus actively contracting with enough power and strength to push your babies through? Your doctor will also be asking about a fourth P—position. Depending on whether your babies are presenting vertex or breech, your doctor will be preparing for a vaginal delivery or C-section.

On to the Delivery Room

Birthing rooms are terrific places, but when it comes to the final portion of a twin birth, I always use a delivery/operating room—just in case something goes wrong. If your doctor also prefers to deliver twins in an operating room, everyone will start preparing for the big move when your first baby's head descends. They'll roll you to the delivery room, sonogram in tow, along with a team of supporting personnel.

Who's in the Delivery Room?

You might be surprised by the large number of people who show up at the eleventh hour. During several hours of labor, you may have had only occasional visits from your doctor and the labor-floor nurses. Then, suddenly, you're attended by what seems like an enormous entourage of medical personnel as noted in Chapter 16, including:

- an anesthesiologist;
- one or two pediatricians—to care for the babies; if your babies are premature, there may be two or more doctors and/or specialists in perinatal (newborn) care;
- one or two nurses—to help both your ob/gyn and the pediatrician(s);
- your support people—father, partner, birth coach, midwife, friends, family, doula;
- resident(s) and interns—there to help out as well as to learn about multiple births.

Some patients find the crowd intimidating or overwhelming; others are so preoccupied with the excitement of delivery that they barely even notice. Either way, rest assured that all these people are necessary backups to ensure your safe, healthy delivery.

When I delivered Luz's twins, she was quite annoyed that she couldn't continue her labor in the birthing room. She was rather put off by the huge crowd present at her delivery, and when she got pregnant a second time, she made me promise that she would be able to finish delivering in the birthing room, with as much privacy as possible.

As it happened, her second pregnancy was a breech presentation. Although I was able to deliver her vaginally, I had to take her to the OR for the breech delivery—and once again, Luz gave birth for the eyes of a watching crowd. Afterward she told me jokingly that although she was grateful for the chance to deliver three healthy babies under my care, she'd never believe me again!

As each baby gets closer to the vaginal opening, your doctor will decide whether there's enough room for the baby's head to emerge. If not, he or she may do an *episiotomy,* a small incision of the perineum to make your vaginal opening larger and allow the baby's head to come out. Without an episiotomy, the baby's head might cause you to tear jaggedly—a laceration that is much harder to repair than the clean, controlled cut of an episiotomy. Ironically, fit, athletic women are more likely to have taut, resistant muscles in the perineum—and are therefore more likely to need this procedure! However, that fitness is very helpful when you're looking for extra stamina and ability to push. Your ob/gyn will restore the muscles in the perineum during the repair of the episiotomy.

On the other hand, in a multiple birth with its smaller fetuses, the perineum may only need to be massaged, so that an episiotomy may not be necessary. Some studies show that healing from minor tears may indeed be preferable.

At this stage, the word *labor* really comes into play. As anyone who's ever delivered a child will tell you, you're going to be working very, very hard. You may feel the uncontrollable urge to push—but your doctor will be guiding you, perhaps advising you to hold off, perhaps urging you to push even harder. If you've taken birth classes, you and your coach will be drawing on everything you've learned—

the breathing exercises, the tricks for sharpening concentration and focus. Around you, the team of nurses, pediatricians, and other medical personnel may be rushing around, preparing for the new arrivals—but you are attuned to the demands of your body and its almost overpowering need to push this baby out into the world.

Under these circumstances, I always find it incredibly moving that the mother giving birth—in the midst of all the pressure, pain, and excitement of those last few minutes—is so willing to rise above the tumult and discomfort and really *listen* to her doctor, as I tell her when to push and when to hold back. Although I've seen it time and time again, I'm always amazed at the way my patients seem to rise above themselves, how despite all obstacles, their whole being seems concentrated on doing what's best for their babies.

Coming Out Headfirst: A Vertex/Vertex Delivery

Ideally, your babies are positioned so that both will come out headfirst. The first baby's head will *crown*—emerging from your vagina, then returning back in as the contraction recedes. Guided by your doctor and your birth coach, you'll be pushing, working hard, but relieved in the knowledge that the head will soon fully emerge, to be followed very quickly by the rest of the baby's body.

If the child is having difficulty emerging, I might perform a *forceps* delivery, using forceps to pull the child out of the womb. *Vacuum extraction,* in which the sucking force of a vacuum helps pull the child out, is another possibility.

Once your baby is out, his or her cord will be clamped, then cut. Ideally, the baby will be handed immediately to your partner, although if there's a medical problem or if the newborn is premature, a pediatrician will begin to care for him or her. If there's no problem, your partner will hold the baby for a few minutes before a nurse dries the child off and swaddles him or her in warm, dry clothes.

You, meanwhile, are hopefully enjoying a few minutes of relief and triumph, and you might even have the chance to hold your first baby before going on to the second delivery. Your ob/gyn will have continued to monitor the progress of Baby B.

Forceps and Vacuum Delivery

These two methods of helping a slow birth along can't be used in every circumstance, but when the conditions are right, these techniques are invaluable. They're especially useful if the mother is too tired to push, if there seems to be little progress in the birth, or if the fetal heartbeat is slowing, suggesting that the baby, too, is getting tired and may soon be going into distress.

It's possible to use forceps or a vacuum extractor when:

- the pelvis is clearly wide enough for the baby that the mother is carrying;
- the baby's head is engaged (at the level of the spine as it moves into the pelvis);
- the anesthesia is adequate (pudendal blocks, a kind of local anesthesia, can be used, as can an epidural);
- the operator is comfortable with the procedure.

A doctor might also use forceps or a vacuum extractor to speed the second delivery when there's a greater risk that the placenta will begin to separate or, most urgently, if the placenta already *has* separated. (The second baby is still receiving blood through the umbilical cord, so if the placenta detaches from the mother, the baby's oxygen supply will be cut off.)

I personally prefer forceps, which is the method that I've been trained in, and I've performed lots of forceps deliveries for twins. With breech extractions, I use Piper forceps, which are extra long, allowing me to reach in and ease out the baby's head, for a less traumatic delivery of the head. Either type of forceps delivery involves little or no trauma to the baby if the forceps are properly used.

Vacuum extractors have recently gotten some bad press, since they've resulted in some cases of *cephalohematoma*—a condition in which blood collects under the baby's scalp. But in the hands of a skilled operator who's comfortable with the procedure, vacuum extraction is a safe and useful method of delivery.

"That time *between* the births—I've never felt anything like it," Zoe says. "I was so thrilled that Nicole was born. And then that whole last part of the birth is so intense. I couldn't believe I was going to go through it all over again."

The average time between deliveries is 17 minutes, but your own time may be only a few minutes—or as long as several hours. In the "old days," we used to believe that it was dangerous to allow more than 30 minutes to elapse between deliveries, for fear that the placenta might separate and put Baby B at risk. Now, with more sophisticated monitoring techniques, most doctors believe it's all right to wait a bit longer.

On the other hand, there is a higher rate of C-sections associated with longer breaks between births, precisely because of the increased risk that the placenta might detach. So if the second birth is taking *too* long, I might order some Pitocin or even perform an amniotomy (if it's a vertex birth) to keep things moving.

As you wait for the second birth, your ob/gyn will give you a pelvic exam to find out how far along you are with Baby B. He or she will also give you a sonogram to find out more about the baby's position, making sure that Baby B is a vertex delivery and that there's no cord prolapse (a situation in which the umbilical cord falls out first—which might result in danger to the baby). Your doctor might attempt an external cephalic version at this point—pushing the baby's head down from the outside, with sonographic guidance.

Assuming that Baby B is also a vertex delivery, if Baby B's head has engaged, I might do an amniotomy—breaking the waters around the second sac—to help move the child along. If I'm doing a breech extraction, I'll grab the baby's feet, do an amniotomy, and then ease the baby out.

Once Baby B is out, his or her cord will also be clamped and cut. A nurse will mark the clamp, so that later your doctor can tell which cord belonged to which twin. (Sometimes, diagnosis of the cords reveals possible problems: If the cord has only two blood vessels instead of three, that might indicate kidney problems or other structural abnormalities. Hopefully, with sonograms and other screening procedures, we'll know about these ahead of time.)

Ideally, Baby B, too, will be handed immediately to the mother's

What's the Percentage?

TYPE OF DELIVERY	PERCENTAGE	RECOMMENDED DELIVERY METHOD
Vertex/vertex	45%	Vaginal
Vertex/breech or Vertex/transverse	35–40%	Attempt a vaginal delivery if it meets the criteria
Breech/vertex or Breech/breech	15–20%	C-section

partner (Baby A may already have been tested, checked out, cleaned up, and be ready to hand to the mother). Once again, a pediatrician and nurse will be standing by, reading to provide postpartum care for Baby B if needed.

"When I saw Jack standing there holding both of my boys, it was probably the proudest moment in my life," Marsha says simply. "Nothing I've ever done has ever been such a thrill."

"I was so relieved it was all finally over, I felt like crying," Rosario recalls. "I'm not sure *what* I felt—there was just this huge flood of tears."

"I just kept thinking, '*We did it! We did it!*'" Jeannette says. "And when I was holding both babies, and they were *mine,* and I was a *mother*—I felt like my whole life had turned upside down and inside out. But in a good way."

Heads and Feet: A Vertex/Breech Delivery

What if Baby A comes out headfirst, but Baby B presents with feet or bottom? As I've mentioned before, I might perform an external cephalic version (manipulating the mother's abdomen to help push the baby's head down).

The longer we wait for the second birth, the greater the risk of placental abruption. So if the baby is presenting feet first, I'd probably do a *breech extraction:* I'd reach inside the mother, grab the baby's little feet, and pull the child out feet first. I'd want to complete this maneuver as soon as possible after the first birth, to take advantage of the fact that the mother's cervix is still fully dilated. Then I'd do an amniotomy—rupture the membranes surrounding the baby. I'd be very careful not to do that latter procedure, however, until the baby's feet were firmly in my hands.

If the baby is presenting tush first, I'd reach in and push the tush out of the way so that I could grab the baby's feet, or else I'd wait until the baby had descended a bit farther, do an amniotomy, and deliver as a *frank breech*—an assisted breech delivery.

In all cases of breech birth, of course, we'd be monitoring the baby closely. If there is any problem, any sign of fetal distress, we'd move right to an emergency C-section to deliver Twin B.

You may have heard of some very rare cases of *asynchronous* twin births—births in which the twins are born a few days or even a few weeks apart. This is a heroic and extreme measure, however, and is performed only in cases of extreme prematurity, when the benefits to the baby of remaining inside the mother are judged to outweigh the enormous risk of infection to both mother and baby. Obviously, this procedure is only possible if the amniotic membranes of the remaining babies are still intact. Usually in these cases, the remaining babies would be tested for infection by doing an amniocentesis and checking the amniotic fluid for bacteria and other signs of infection.

If such heroic measures are taken, the cord of the baby who's delivered is sutured near the cervix, so that the placenta can continue to nourish the remaining baby or babies. In a recent case of triplets at our hospital, for example, Baby A was born prematurely and, sadly, died. However, Babies B and C were able to remain in the womb for a while longer—and, when they were born, they survived and thrived.

The Third Stage of Labor: Delivery of the Placenta

After both babies have been delivered, the third stage of labor begins: delivery of the placenta. In a twin birth, the placenta usually weighs close to a pound and a half—a good deal of material for your uterus to expel. As a result, you may feel cramps similar to those you felt during birth. While your contractions continue, your doctor will hold the umbilical cords and gently guide the placenta through your birth canal. In some cases, your doctor will reach in and remove the placenta by hand.

Either way, delivery of the placenta usually takes only five or ten minutes. Afterward, your uterus will be vigorously massaged to help the contractions continue, which will in turn help you cut down on blood loss. You might also be given more Pitocin through your IV or possibly an injection of prostaglandin or Methergine.

"You had to give me Pitocin *again*," Miriam remembers. "And then you were massaging my uterus to help, and by that point, I was *so* ready to be done with the whole birth thing. I couldn't wait to hold my children, to start nursing, to start getting to know them."

"I actually felt kind of sad," Luz admits. "Not that I liked being pregnant, exactly. And not that I wasn't glad to have my babies. But there was something about the whole thing being over . . ."

Once delivery *is* over, your ob/gyn will examine the inside of your vagina to make sure that no rips or tears continue to bleed. You'll also get a rectal exam, to make sure that your rectal sphincter (the ring-shaped muscles that allow you to contract your anus) are intact and to check for any vaginal tearing that might have extended into the rectum. If you did have an episiotomy, now is when you'll be sutured, with stitches that your body will absorb in time.

Finally, your ob/gyn will examine the placenta. Examining the placental membranes helps confirm zygosity (whether your twins are "fraternal"/dizygotic or "identical"/monozygotic)—information that you'll need for many reasons, particularly if your babies have medical problems later in life. Your doctor will also examine the twins' umbilical cords to make sure that they have three blood vessels rather than two. If you have decided to bank your babies' cord blood (see Chapter 12), this is when your doctor will harvest it.

The Problematic Apgar

If your twins emerge with medical problems, they will probably be whisked away for immediate neonatal care. If they come out safe and healthy, they will probably be given to you and your partner to hold while an *Apgar score* is calculated.

Apgar tests are given at 1, 5, and sometimes 10 or 15 minutes after birth. The test is used to make sure that the baby is doing well and to identify any problem that needs special treatment. The Apgar features five categories, each of which is worth two points:

- heart rate;
- rate of breathing;
- skin color;
- muscle tone;
- reflex reactions (known as *reflex irritability*).

A perfect Apgar, obviously, is 10, but in actual fact, the best one-minute Apgar that any baby can get is 9, since all babies are born with *acrocyanosis*—that is, with blue feet and hands.

In any case, the relevancy of the Apgar test is somewhat controversial. The procedure was first developed in 1953 as a way of determining which newborns needed special attention—and it's still considered effective toward that end. However, over the years, doctors and patients have tended to see the Apgar as a predictor of future neurological problems—though in fact there's relatively little clinical evidence that this test can be used that way.

In the diagnosis of cerebral palsy, for example, the one-minute Apgar has no predictive power whatsoever. Even among babies whose five-minute Apgar score is 3 or lower, only 5 percent prove to have cerebral palsy. Persistently low 10- and 15-minute Apgars have slightly more relevance, but they are still fairly unreliable. Even when we know that a baby has suffered from asphyxia (the inability to breathe) at birth, that's not necessarily a predictor of the baby's future condition. A baby with a difficult birth or an extremely low Apgar can easily have a full recovery—so don't take a low score too seriously.

Most pediatricians agree that the Apgar is even less relevant in the case of preterm babies. So if your twins were born early, your doctors will be testing them in other ways.

Looking Ahead

Congratulations! You're now the proud mother of twins! The final chapters of this book will help you know what to expect in your first few days of multiple parenthood (Chapter 18) and how to cope with your new responsibilities (Chapter 19).

18.

"They're Here!": What Happens
When Your Twins Arrive

❧

You've made it through pregnancy. You've made it through labor. You have two beautiful babies whom you'll soon be taking home. What happens now?

In this chapter, I'll talk you through the postpartum period, from the first few minutes of holding your children to the first few days in the hospital. For more on longer-term issues, see the next chapter.

For most women, this is a time of intense ups and downs: wonder at the miracle of your new babies, a feeling of being overwhelmed at having *two* new lives to care for, amazement that these two babies are now *outside* your body, relief at the end of pregnancy, joy in the two new human beings who are yours to love and enjoy. You may also experience mild or severe postpartum depression or, at the very least, a sense of disorientation as you get reacquainted with a new body in which *everything* seems different—hormonal activity, body shape, appetite, emotions, energy levels.

"I was all over the place," Natalie recalls. "I would lie there in my hospital bed, just weeping—I didn't even know why, I was just so overwhelmed. Then the nurse would bring the babies in and I'd be there with Janet and our children, and I would feel so calm and peaceful, like nothing would ever matter as much as just this moment. Then Janet and the babies would leave, and all I'd want to do was sleep. The roller coaster just went on and on."

"I expected to love my children," Miriam says, "but I had no idea how *much*. I'd be in the middle of all that busy-ness—feeding them and changing them and finding out that we didn't have something I needed and calling Ira to come get it for me—and then I'd look down at them, and I'd think, 'Wow. I'm their *mother*.' "

In this period as in all others, you'll find yourself balancing two opposite approaches: On the one hand, you've done your homework (including reading this book!), so you have some idea of what to expect. On the other hand, you'll realize again and again that however much you know, you are always going to be profoundly surprised, by your children and by yourself—a condition that can easily last for 20 years or more. Welcome to multiple parenthood!

Facing the Postpartum Period

You and your twins will probably need to stay in the hospital for two to five days, depending on what kind of delivery you had or if there were any complications. Your stay will be shorter for a vaginal delivery without complications, longer for a C-section.

If you carried your twins to term and there were no complications, they'll probably be ready to go home when you are. If you had a C-section or a complicated birth, they may be ready to go home *before* you are. Premature twins may need to stay in the hospital for a few extra days or weeks, depending on their gestational age (how many weeks they spent in the womb). (For more on premature twins, see page 294.)

"Actually, one of the good parts of having a C-section was getting to stay in the hospital," Natalie admits. "I would have thought I'd want to go right home, but honestly, it was such an overwhelming change, I was kind of glad to be someplace where other people were taking care of me."

"Because they came at thirty weeks, both our kids had to spend some time in intensive care," Shana recalls. "I'd go visit them and nurse them, and that was wonderful—and then I had to give them back to the people in NICU [neonatal intensive-care unit], and that was awful. But we got through it."

"I was torn, frankly," says Zoe. "I really couldn't wait to get back to Sean and Lissa and my house, and of course I was glad that both our twins were doing well. At the same time, I must admit, the idea of taking care of *four* children all of a sudden—it was a little much."

One of the most difficult parts of adjusting to the postpartum period is the recognition that you're going to need time—at least six weeks—before you're back to your old, prepregnancy levels of health and energy. If you had a C-section, your recovery period may well be longer. But even if you delivered vaginally, without complications, your body will need time to recuperate from the hard, intense work of a multiple pregnancy and labor. Women who have given birth before, or who have been close to other mothers, may be surprised at how much longer it takes to recover from a multiple pregnancy. Remember that every woman's body is unique, and give yourself all the time you need.

"I *thought* by the time I had Nicole and Nick Junior, I'd finally accepted that *this* pregnancy was different from the other two," says Zoe. "But no. I was still surprised at how much harder it was to come back from this one—especially because you don't know what tired is until you've breast-fed *two* babies!"

If you did have a cesarean, be sure to notice any redness or swelling around your incision, which could indicate infection. Your doctor will let you know about caring for your wound. Some women are sent home before their sutures or staples are removed; others have everything taken care of before they leave the hospital.

After they've given birth, many women start thinking about losing the rest of their pregnancy weight as quickly as possible. I urge you to resist that temptation, at least for the first few months. Even if you're not nursing your twins, your body needs lots of energy to cope both with your recovery and with the demands of two new babies. And if you're nursing, you'll need a well-balanced diet that includes lots of protein, calcium, and fluids to produce milk for your twins. By the way, you are burning off 500 kilocalories a day per baby if you're breast-feeding.

Recent studies show that it can take up to 12 weeks after you deliver for some of the cardiovascular changes caused by your pregnancy to return to "normal." So focus on healing, recovering, and getting whatever sleep you can possibly manage—and give yourself a break over the weight.

"Actually, by the time we finally brought the twins home, I was so relieved that they were all right, I wasn't even thinking about my weight anymore," Shana admits. "And by the time I *was* thinking about it again, I had already lost more than half of those pregnancy pounds—because of the nursing, I guess."

Getting Used to Your New Body

As soon as you deliver, your body starts to adjust to its new role. You'll notice this change in lots of little ways, but perhaps the most dramatic is in how fluids shift and rebalance, pretty much from the moment that the babies leave your body.

The first thing you'll notice is the way edema, or swelling, decreases in your limbs and face as your body begins to lose the extra fluids that it no longer needs. You'll probably pass more urine and urinate more often—and you're likely to be quite thirsty as a result. Be sure to drink lots of water, juice, milk, Gatorade, and other healthy fluids, just as you did during pregnancy. Sometime in the initial few days you may notice a bit more swelling of your feet as your body's fluids return to normal.

You'll probably also notice some heavy bleeding right after birth—even heavier than your heaviest period. This bloody vaginal discharge is known as *lochia*. Don't be alarmed if you have to change your sanitary napkin every few hours. Most women bleed for several weeks after they give birth, so keep taking your iron supplements and, again, drink lots of water.

➤ ALERT: If you're passing blood clots or huge amounts of blood, or if you've got a fever, let your doctor know right away.

In the first few hours after delivery, your overdistended uterus will be shrinking down to its normal size, and you may experience some painful contractions as a result. Talk to your ob/gyn about what you can do to manage the pain, keeping in mind that if you're nursing you'll be limited in what kind of medication you can take. Medication at this point might also make you constipated. You can, however, use cold packs that fit onto your sanitary napkin (the nurse may have given you one right after delivery), which help combat the soreness in your vaginal and rectal areas.

What to Bring to the Hospital . . .

One of my patients has a special message for other multiple moms. "When you go to the hospital," she says, "be sure to bring a big box of superplus sanitary pads. The hospital will give you menstrual pads, but they're useless, frankly, because they're so small. And the hospital pads come with those little belts, which are just ridiculous. Bring your own pads—the kind that have adhesive on the bottom so they can attach to your panties."

One common problem at this stage is hemorrhoids. That's because your pregnancy-dilated veins take time to return to normal. For your own comfort and to allow the normal receding of the dilated veins, avoid constipation (drink plenty of fluids and stay on your fiber-rich diet!), and if necessary use hemorrhoid creams or suppositories, such as Anusol. Tucks or another brand of witch-hazel pad can also provide relief for itchy or uncomfortable areas. Sitz baths can help—run yourself a low tub of tepid water to soak in, but no soap, please—some women find that soap or bubble bath can irritate those itchy areas.

The Breast versus the Bottle: Making the Decision

Breast- versus bottle-feeding is a tough decision for many mothers, especially where multiples are concerned. There are lots of factors to take into account—even more than for the mothers of singletons.

The first factor I'd urge you to consider is whether your children are premature or full-term. If they're premature, there are many compelling reasons to breast-feed, at least for the first weeks. We know that breast-fed babies generally have fewer allergies and that their immune systems are stronger, providing them with more protection against infection. These are advantages that might make a great deal of difference to premature infants, in addition to the fact that infants generally tolerate breast milk better than formula—giving your undersize new-borns a crucial advantage in their early efforts to gain weight.

It's also true that breast-feeding offers a unique opportunity for bonding. If your premature children are in the NICU, you and they might appreciate that special feeding time, when you're giving them something that can come only from *you*. It can be hard to see your tiny newborns being cared for by doctors, nurses, and specialists, surrounded by the elaborate medical technology of a modern hospital (however grateful we all are to that technology for saving lives that might once have been lost). If you have the chance to breast-feed your infants, you have the satisfaction of knowing that you're providing a kind of care that even the highly trained neonatal staff can't match. Fortunately, most NICUs encourage parents to breast-feed, so if you do make this decision, you can expect the staff's support.

It's especially important to breast-feed infants if you have a family history of allergies, if your previous children have developed asthma, if your previous children had trouble digesting formula, or if there's a family history of diabetes. In all of these cases, breast-feeding can provide significant benefits to combat the family health problems, and you should make every effort to give your children the medical advantages of breast milk if you can.

What if your infants are full-term and you have none of these medical problems? Well, in the ideal world, you'd probably still be better off breast-feeding: It's the ideal food for your children, it offers a special time for bonding, it leads to less indigestion and colic—and it saves lots of money! It also frees you from having to lug bottles, formulas, and all the other feeding paraphernalia with you on a trip to the park or to a friend's house, which, when you're packing and carrying equipment for two, is quite a savings of time, energy, and weight. And speaking of weight, you'll certainly burn off those extra pregnancy pounds a lot more quickly if you're nursing.

On the other hand, if you're breast-feeding two infants, you'll be feeding them every two to three hours when they're small, which means that as soon as you've gotten them both fed and changed, it's just about time to start feeding them again. That's a huge commitment—and it's not necessarily one that you'll be able or willing to make, given your responsibilities to your job, your other children, your partner, and yourself. As you make this important decision, here are some factors you'll probably have to weigh:

- **Did you deliver vaginally or by C-section?** A vaginal delivery will probably leave you with a bit more energy and a somewhat faster recovery than a C-section. If you're recovering from a C-section—and coping with some residual pain from the incision—it may be more difficult to consider breast-feeding.

- **How is your health?** Depending on your age and physical condition (including any medications you are taking), you might indeed have the energy to nurse—or you might find yourself too exhausted even to consider it. Be realistic about your limits—there is more than one way to feed your children, but you are the only mother they've got!

- **What kind of household help do you have?** Ideally, you have a partner, friends, relatives, and maybe even an au pair or someone for hire who can do all the *non*-breast-feeding chores around the house—but, as we've said, this is far from an ideal world. You may also prefer to share the special time of feeding with your partner and with trusted friends and relatives.

- **What's your work situation?** Breast-feeding twins and working full-time is a real challenge. Remember, when your twins are small, they may need to be fed every two to three hours. Even if you supplement actual breast-feeding with bottle-fed breast milk, that's a lot of time at the breast pump. Basically, breast-feeding twins *is* a full-time job, at least for the first few months. It may be difficult to combine this commitment with any other ongoing responsibility.

- **How do you and your partner want to divide up the household work?** The great advantage of bottle-feeding, of course, is that your partner can share in the work—and the bonding. You don't have to take *every* nighttime feeding, and both of you may be more comfortable when you have similar roles. On the other hand, if you *are* breast-feeding, there are plenty of other ways for your children and your partner to bond. Giving the children their bath, changing their diapers, or simply playing with them, holding them, and cuddling them are all perfectly good ways to bond.

- **How do you feel about bonding with your twins?** One of the challenges of having twins is that it often feels as though there's never enough time with either one. My patients who breast-feed tell me that they appreciate the special nursing time that allows them to focus on each twin separately. (Of course, some of my patients breast-feed both twins simultaneously—which certainly is more time-effective than bottle-feeding!) But that first year of twin infancy is such a jumble, with so many new demands and so little sleep, that it's nice to have some special "quiet time" with your children.
- **Are there any older children in your household?** It can be hard for children to understand that babies have special needs. Somehow breast-feeding—as opposed to bottle-feeding—makes it extra clear, even to toddlers, that Mom just *has* to spend time feeding the babies, since obviously, only *she* can breast-feed.
- **What "middle ground" is there?** Some women manage to combine breast-feeding with bottle-feeding, either by pumping breast milk or by using formula to supplement the breast-feeding. That way, they can involve their partners in those crucial night feedings or feel more free about leaving the house for a brief errand or even to go to work.

It's a powerful experience to nurse multiples. It gives you a greater respect for the wonders of the human body—that by yourself you can supply milk for two, three, or four babies. And it's an amazing feeling to know that you're giving something to your children that only *you* can provide (wet nurses having fallen out of favor!).

I myself breast-fed my first and fourth daughters and bottle-fed my twins. I knew I was going back to work five weeks after they came, and I wanted us to all settle in comfortably to a bottle-feeding routine rather than having to deal with weaning them and going back to work at the same time. Although I loved the special bonding time of breast-feeding my other two, I must say that I also loved my husband's greater involvement in feeding our twins. (Jim and I decided to keep a "feeding log" to make sure that *both* twins were indeed getting fed!)

As with pretty much every decision involved in parenting twins,

The Breast versus the Bottle: The Great Debate

Miriam: "Breast-feed *two* babies? No way! I wanted to feel like a mother, not like a cow!"

Sarah: "I wish I *could* have breast-fed my babies. But since there were three of them, I was afraid that I really wouldn't have been able to handle the physical strain, let alone the time commitment."

Jeannette: "I was eager to get back to work as soon as possible. But I also really believed in breast-feeding—I'd read about how good those first few days were for the babies and about how it helped with bonding, and, frankly, I wanted to know what it felt like. So I compromised—I breast-fed for six weeks, which seemed to take care of the basic nutritional part of it, and then I weaned them, which was awful and wrenching, but it did mean I could go back to work. I'm glad I did it that way, finally, because I know I was a much better mother working than I would have been staying home all day."

Natalie: "I was very committed to breast-feeding. I had planned to take that first year to stay home with my children, so there was no conflict with work or anything like that. I think I got much closer to each one of them—there's something about the nursing experience that just isn't like anything else."

Zoe: "I had breast-fed both Sean and Lissa, and I was really committed to giving it a try with the twins. It was kind of overwhelming—but in a funny way, I think it was reassuring to my older kids, besides helping me bond with the babies. Breast-feeding the babies made it so clear to my other kids that *these* were the babies, and *they* were the big kids. And nobody but Mommy could feed the babies. I think that made it easier for Sean, especially, to understand why I *had* to spend so much time with the little ones."

you and your partner will have to figure out what's best for you. What worked for you in a previous singleton pregnancy, or what's worked for your friends and relatives who have singletons, just might not fit your new situation. Breast-feeding is a great gift to your babies if it's doable—but, depending on your situation, it may not be. So give yourself a break. This first year is going to involve a lot of compromise on everybody's part, and compromise is always easier when you don't expect yourself to be Supermom.

If You Nurse Your Twins . . .

Fairly soon after you deliver, you'll probably be feeding your twins. If your twins are born without complications, they'll be ready to suck, whether bottle or breast. You, however, may need some time to get used to the sensation! If your babies were born full-term, you may be surprised at how vigorous their suck reflex is; if your babies were just a bit premature, you'll be astonished at how quickly they catch up.

Be ready to experiment with different positions as you hold your suckling children, and know that your nipples will need some time to adjust. Some women say that labor was a snap compared to nursing! Keep soothing lanolin cream by your bedside to use after your feedings, and be patient with yourself.

Some women seem to have trouble producing milk at first. The more your babies nurse, the more milk you're likely to produce, so don't give up. Your supply of milk will eventually grow to match the demand. And don't worry about your babies not getting enough nourishment. The hospital staff will be weighing your babies frequently. If they see any cause for concern, they'll talk to you about supplementing your nursing with a bottle or two.

Of course, when you get your babies home, you'll want to watch out for the signs of dehydration and malnourishment. Your babies should be producing six to eight wet diapers a day: Check with your doctor if they're not. Their skin should be moist and somewhat shiny. If they're excessively restless or excessively lethargic, that might also signal a problem.

Nursing Hygiene

Your babies suck milk through your nipples—more specifically, through the many little openings in your nipples, which dilate as they release milk. These openings don't only let milk out; they may also let bacteria in. Guard against infection by rinsing your breasts between

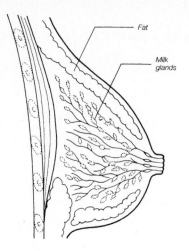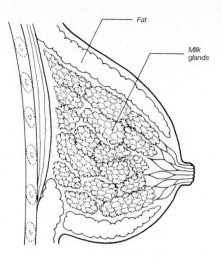

Before pregnancy   During pregnancy

FIGURE 1

feedings, first with warm soapy water, then with clear water—your babies will hate the taste of soap! (See Figure 1.)

You should also wash your hands frequently, before and after nursing, especially when you have a cold. Don't let your hands touch your nipple or your baby's mouth until you've washed.

If an infection does enter through your nipples, you might get *mastitis,* a painful condition accompanied by fever, chills, muscle aches, and an overall feeling of illness and fatigue. If you think you're sick, tell your doctor right away. Your doctor will probably prescribe antibiotics that are nursing-safe. Warm showers a couple of times daily, warm compresses, and regularly emptying your breasts are important too.

One other possible infection is *thrush,* a fungal growth that can affect both your nipples and your babies' mouths. If you notice that either your nipples or their mouths are red and inflamed, and/or if your babies' tongues are white and coated, this may be a sign of thrush. Your doctor can give you a topical antifungal cream to help clear up the problem on your breasts; your babies will be treated separately. One result of thrush can be clogged milk ducts, so again, pump your breasts, use warm compresses, and take warm showers to help your milk continue to flow.

Nursing Patterns

The first liquid that comes from your breasts is known as *colostrum*. You may have had some leakage before delivery and you'll be producing this liquid for the first 48 hours after giving birth. Colostrum may be the most important liquid that your babies ever drink, for it is full of proteins that will support their immune systems.

As you continue to nurse, you'll probably notice your breasts getting markedly bigger—and, possibly, somewhat painful. Some women feel only a slight pressure as feeding time approaches; others find the pressure to be more intense. The sound of a crying baby—their own or someone else's—often causes their milk to "let down." In your first few days of nursing, you'll probably be feeding each baby for about 15 minutes per breast every few hours—a time you'll find yourself anticipating as your breasts tingle and the pressure of the milk grows.

Don't let your breasts become overfull, or *engorged*. An engorged breast feels almost as hard as a rock—and it really hurts! If your breasts and your babies aren't on the same schedule, you may need to release some milk with a breast pump, or express some milk by hand when you're in the shower. (For more on breast pumps and storing milk, see Chapter 19.)

You'll probably want to time each baby at the breast, to make sure each one is getting enough nourishment—but not staying at the breast too long! Babies are efficient little machines, and it takes one only a few minutes to empty your breast of milk; after that, he or she is sucking primarily for comfort. If you limit your initial nursing times to only 10 or 15 minutes per breast, you'll give your nipples time to toughen up and lower the risk of the tiny cuts that can introduce infection.

Nourishing Yourself

If you are breast-feeding, make sure you're getting 400 to 500 extra calories a day per baby. Also be sure to drink 8 to 12 cups of fluid a day. There are lots of folk remedies that explain how to boost milk production. One of my favorites is brewer's yeast, which is rich in B vitamins and good for relaxation as well as an energy boost.

If You're Bottle-Feeding...

If you're feeding your children by bottle instead of by breast, you might want to skim the preceding section to get some idea of your babies' feeding patterns, as well as to find out how your breasts may feel until they "learn" that they won't be nursing. I suggest that you wear a somewhat binding bra, such as a jogging bra, until your milk production stops. If your breasts are stimulated, they'll probably release milk—and the more milk they release, the more milk they'll produce.

It's also important to maintain good hygiene when you—or anyone else—bottle-feeds your babies. Make sure anyone feeding your twins washes his or her hands, to guard against infection. Sometimes it's hard to remember how little and new your babies are. An infection that a healthy adult could resist or shake off becomes an overpowering assault on an infant whose immune system is not yet fully developed.

We once thought babies' bottles had to be sterilized. Now we know better—but it's still important to keep the bottles clean and to wash them after every feeding. Don't use a bottle for more than one feeding without washing it first. And don't let a bottle sit in your fridge after a feeding and then use it again—wash out every bottle after every feeding. (Mothers who advocate breast-feeding like to point out the time-consuming nature of washing and rewashing all those bottles.) Try not to get overwhelmed by all the bottle-related chores, though. Accepting the many limits on their time is a lesson that parents keep learning again and again.

Feeding Your Twins: When There Are Complications

As we've seen, full-term babies are born knowing how to suck, whether they have a human or a rubber nipple in their mouths. Some premature babies are also born with a strong suck reflex, while others—even those born later—have to learn this response outside of the womb. Babies born past 34 weeks, however, usually *can* learn to suck, swallow, and breathe, and so they, like full-term infants, can be fed right after birth.

But some babies, usually those born before 34 weeks, are not fed right away. If your twins are among these and you want to breast-feed, you'll have to use a breast pump during this time; otherwise, your milk might dry up. The hospital will probably have a breast pump for you to use and will then feed your newborns colostrum and breast milk by tube. "It was kind of an odd feeling, starting with that breast pump instead of with the babies at my breast," Shana recalls. "But I really wanted to nurse, so I was grateful that the technology was available."

If your premature babies can't nurse yet, you'll probably have to pump your breasts at least six to eight times a day. A pump with a double setup allows you to pump both breasts at once—saving you a few precious waking hours.

My own feeling is that if you're committed to breast-feeding, you'll definitely need a breast pump—and it should probably be a full-size electric one, expensive as they are. The hand pumps or mini-electric ones just don't work as well, and if you're breast-feeding twins, you'll want to save every ounce of time, patience, and energy that you can. If you can't afford to buy the more expensive pump, you can rent one—and I promise you, you'll be glad you did. ("We rented an electric twin breast pump," Rosario recalls, "and it saved my life. I used to tell my husband that the only reason I got in a ten-minute shower each day was because the pump could work on both breasts at the same time.")

Sometimes, even if children *can* suck, they can't suck long enough or hard enough to nourish themselves properly. In that case, you'll need a breast pump to empty your breasts—both to keep your milk coming in and to feed it to your children.

Generally, even premature babies can nurse within a few days of birth, even if they're only able to do so once a day. I recommend to nursing mothers that they try to breast-feed at least once a day as early as possible. Gradually, they can replace bottle- or tube-feeding with more frequent sessions of breast-feeding.

When Your Twins Are Premature: Less Than 34 Weeks

One of the remarkable achievements of modern medicine is our new ability to keep alive babies born between 24 and 34 weeks of gestation. This increased survival rate has taught us something else: There is virtually no difference in survival or complication rates between twins and singletons born at the same age and at similar birth weight.

So if your babies were born prematurely, take heart. Almost 80 percent of all children born between 24 and 31 weeks survive—and the rates are going up all the time. And most of the death rates during this period are caused by extremely low birth weights (babies weighing less than one kilogram—two pounds—at birth). Our new increased survival rates are due to the prenatal use of steroids, which help the babies' lungs manufacture surfactant and so mature while they're still in the womb, and to the use of surfactant in the newborns, which allows the lungs to expand and stay open.

Coping with Respiratory Distress Syndrome

As we saw in Chapter 15, one of the biggest problems faced by premature babies is their immature lungs. When a baby's lungs aren't mature enough to allow the child to breathe adequately, he or she suffers from *respiratory distress syndrome,* or RDS. Male babies are more prone to RDS than females, since their lungs don't seem to mature as quickly.

Technically speaking, RDS is caused by the lack of surfactant, so the development of synthetic surfactant has brought about a major drop in infant mortality. All but the mildest RDS cases are now treated with surfactant as well as with nutritional support for newborns.

The symptoms of RDS may be relatively mild—or quite severe. Treatment varies accordingly. Babies with mild cases of RDS get humidified oxygen. The next step up is to create "continuous positive airway pressure" (CPAP) by inserting a tube in the baby's nose and pumping oxygen through it. Babies with the most serious cases of RDS are attached to a ventilator via a tube in the windpipe.

Bronchopulmonary Dysplasia

Babies born at less than 28 weeks' gestation have a 50 percent chance of developing *bronchopulmonary dysplasia* (BPD), a chronic lung disease. The earlier the babies were born, the more likely they are to contract BPD.

The good news is that it is possible to recover completely from BPD. The lungs of even normal children take about two years to develop all their airways and passages, and, of course, as the child grows, so does his or her lung capacity. Over the course of this development, a child has the chance to "grow out of" BPD and attain fully normal breathing capacity well before childhood is over.

Apnea

There are many forms of apnea, a temporary interruption in breathing that may plague both children and adults. (You may have heard about sleep apnea, in which adults temporarily stop breathing during sleep.) Many babies born before 34 weeks are at risk for this condition, which may appear as a minor breathing disruption lasting no more than a few seconds at a time or as a major interruption that lasts for 20 seconds or more and is associated with a slowing of the heart rate known as *bradycardia,* usually due to airway obstruction.

Apnea is not a disease in and of itself but rather can be the result of a wide variety of disorders, so if either of your children has apnea, your doctor will try to find the cause. Theophylline or caffeine therapy may be used to treat your babies, as well as nasal CPAP (continuous positive airway pressure).

If a child remains free of apnea for five to seven days, doctors will usually stop medication but continue observation. Sometimes the apnea recurs—and treatment is resumed.

If one or both of your children have apnea, you may be able to bring them home, but you will probably need to invest in a home apnea monitor, which is fairly expensive. Sometimes this device is covered by insurance, or you may be able to get some kind of government assistance. I've known hospitals, home health-care agencies, and even

If You Do Home Monitoring for Apnea, You'll Need:

- **A complete understanding of the diagnosis.** Make sure your doctor explains clearly the symptoms you should be watching for, and the length of time you can expect to monitor your twins.
- **A full understanding of the treatment.** Home monitoring offers many potential benefits, but it's also a risky business. It's not foolproof—and if a problem, or a death, takes place under *your* care, that may be even harder to bear than if the same tragedy happened at the hospital. Home monitoring also requires a level of constancy that may be difficult for two parents—as opposed to a full-time hospital staff—particularly if one parent is at work full-time or if there are other children at home.
- **A good support system.** Can you train family members, baby-sitters, and other caregivers in the use of the monitor? Are your support people ready to take on that responsibility? Hospitals have staffs that monitor in shifts—do you have people to help you and your partner cope with the strain?
- **Lots of serenity and patience.** Home monitoring means that your twins are being monitored every moment of their lives—when they're sleeping, when they're in a car, when they're left alone for a few moments in their high chair or playpen. Some adult must always be listening for the alarm—from the other room, from the front seat, from the depths of sleep. It's also important to know the difference between a true alarm, which indicates that one or both children have stopped breathing, and the (perhaps terrifying) beeping that occurs simply because a monitor's lead has become detached from your baby's skin.
- **An emergency medical plan.** If the monitor does go off, you, your partner, and any other caregivers will need to spring into action. You'll need to have the names and numbers of hospital staff, a plan to get to the hospital, and information about what you can do in the meantime.

medical rental companies to make surprising deals to parents of twins, triplets, and quads, so if you want to do home monitoring, be creative and assertive as you search for a workable arrangement.

In addition to monitoring your twins, you may need to give them medication: typically caffeine, once a day, or aminophylline, which stimulates respiration, three or four times a day.

My patient Larissa gave birth to a boy and a girl at 28 weeks. The boy's breathing patterns were fine, but the girl, Sonya, had apnea. When it came time to take her son, Alex, home from the hospital, Sonya was still being treated for apnea. For a while, Larissa considered treating her daughter at home, but she finally decided that wouldn't be fair to Alex. With regret, Larissa decided to let the hospital staff care for Sonya. "I hated leaving her behind," Larissa said, "and if it had been just her, I wouldn't have done it that way. But I didn't want Alex to be neglected, and if something bad had happened to Sonya while I was with Alex, I would never have forgiven myself. Leaving Sonya in the hospital seemed to be the only way."

Cardiovascular Problems

Every human who's out of the womb must have a means for circulating blood through the lungs, so that the blood can be *oxygenated*. When your babies are still inside you, however, *you* are oxygenating their blood. So your unborn babies' blood bypasses their lungs via an essential fetal blood vessel known as the *ductus arteriosus,* which helps blood move directly from the aorta into the fetal pulmonary (lung) artery.

When a healthy baby is born, this duct closes within 24 hours, so that the newborn's blood can move through the lungs, as it's supposed to do. In some premature babies, however, this duct doesn't close. As a result, the baby has no way to get oxygen into the blood.

This problem is known as PDA, for *patent ductus arteriosus.* It affects some 10 to 20 percent of all premature babies with respiratory distress syndrome and some 30 percent of all babies born at less than 1,500 grams (3⅓ pounds). About 20 percent of the babies affected suffer from immediate hypoxia, or shortage of oxygen, which can affect the brain, threatening the baby's development and, eventually, his or her life. Indocin, or indomethacin, whose antiprostaglandin effect helps correct the problem, may be needed. In some cases, surgery is called for.

Intraventricular Hemorrhage (IVH)

This disability—bleeding within the brain—occurs in 20 to 30 percent of all babies born before 34 weeks and among 50 percent of all very low-birth-weight babies. It also poses a risk of infection in low-birth-weight babies.

Fortunately, IVH rarely causes severe or long-term damage. Only the most severe type, known as "grade IV," causes long-term problems, possibly including seizures. Usually, an ultrasound of the baby's head reveals how severe this problem is and whether there are likely to be any ongoing results from it.

Necrotizing Enterocolitis (NEC)

Some premature infants suffer from this inflammation of the intestine, whose cause is unknown. Early breast-feeding seems to help prevent the condition, however, which is yet another reason why breast-feeding is recommended to the mothers of premature babies. Infants with NEC may risk a perforated intestine and the resulting sepsis (infection). The recommended treatment is to try to drain the bowels, to attack infections with antibiotics, or, if other treatments fail, to resect the affected bowel in a surgical procedure. The prognosis is best when only a small amount of bowel is involved.

Retinopathy of Prematurity (ROP)

Although many premature babies are born with this type of retinal damage, few experience any serious loss of vision as a result. Retinopathy used to be a very common disorder in premature babies. It's caused by increased blood vessels in the retina leading to scarring, retinal detachment, and blindness. We once thought this condition was caused by the high levels of oxygen to which premies were exposed as part of their treatment. Now, with premies surviving at ever-lower birth weights, we are seeing even more examples of retinopathy—and we realize that its incidence increases as birth weights decrease.

Only 10 percent of the babies born with retinopathy will have severe visual problems. However, another concern is hearing loss, which affects some 2 percent of all babies who survive the neonatal ICU.

Group B Strep

As we saw in Chapter 12, some 30 percent of all women are colonized with Group B strep, which lives in the vagina. If this condition was active at the time of delivery, if it was undiagnosed, and if the mother had a vaginal delivery, the babies who passed through the infected area may themselves become infected. Premature babies are especially prone to infections of all kinds, so they should be tested for Group B strep if they show signs of infection. Antibiotics are frequently prescribed in this case.

When Your Twins Are Premature: 34 to 40 Weeks

Time in the Incubator

If your twins were born between 34 and 40 weeks, they're unlikely to have any of the severe problems we've just discussed. However, they may have some difficulty maintaining body temperature, particularly right after birth. Sometimes premature newborn twins need some time in a warming bed or incubator—an enclosed bed surrounded by Plexiglas with "portholes" that allow staff and parents to touch and care for the babies. If your children are born early, they may need to spend several hours or even days in the incubator, interspersed with time for you to hold and feed them. Incubator babies can be either breast- or bottle-fed.

"It was always so hard seeing my little babies in that Plexiglas display case," Vanessa says. "That was one time when I was so glad to be breast-feeding—it seemed like giving them the most I could possibly give them."

Jaundice

Another common problem among newborns is jaundice. Some 60 percent of full-term babies become clinically jaundiced during their first week of life. The problem is even more common—and more serious—among premature babies and may be treated somewhat differently.

Jaundice is the end result of a series of complex chemical interactions, beginning with the breakdown of hemoglobin in your unborn babies. The chemicals that result from the broken-down hemoglobin meet other bodily products in the liver, spleen, and bone marrow, and eventually *bilirubin* is formed.

Bilirubin is a fat-soluble yellowish substance that's toxic to the central nervous system. In healthy babies, any bilirubin in the system is metabolized by the liver—just like any other toxin—and expelled through the intestines as waste. Premature babies, however, may have underdeveloped livers, which can't metabolize bilirubin. The unmetabolized bilirubin stays in the baby's system, gradually turning the baby yellow: first the face and eyes, then the trunk, and finally the legs.

If one or both of your twins is jaundiced, the doctor will begin to investigate the cause of the condition. Usually, the elevated bilirubin levels associated with the disease can be brought down by *phototherapy,* exposure to special lights that help the body clear out the bilirubin. If a full-term baby has jaundice, the doctor is unlikely to order this treatment until the yellow color has spread to the baby's legs. Until then, the doctor will monitor the bilirubin but hope that the liver gains strength to clear up the jaundice on its own, as bilirubin levels usually peak after three to five days.

For premature twins, however—especially those born between 34 and 37 weeks—the doctor may prescribe phototherapy as soon as the yellow color reaches the baby's belly. Your doctor will also be keeping track of your baby's bilirubin count—the amount of bilirubin per deciliter of blood. This count plus your babies' clinical condition will determine whether the doctor orders treatment. Most doctors will prescribe treatment if there are 19 or 20 milligrams of bilirubin per deciliter in a premature baby's blood; some will order phototherapy at 15 mg/dl to keep levels from rising any higher. The goal of all this treatment is to avoid *kernicterus,* the yellow staining of the nerve cells, which can result in damage to the central nervous system.

My patient Mickie gave birth to a boy and a girl at 32 weeks. The girl seemed to be doing fine, but the boy had jaundice, which was a special concern because he had been born so early. I prescribed phototherapy for him fairly soon, and slowly he began to recover. His sister, meanwhile, was spending time in the incubator, monitored closely because of her young age. "At least they both had to be in the hospital," Mickie says. "I don't know what I would have done if Max had had to stay while Mara came home."

Phototherapy

If your twins do need phototherapy, they'll be placed under a bank of fluorescent lights, either in the hospital or at home. Blood will be taken regularly to monitor their bilirubin counts, so if you're treating them at home, you may need to learn to do this too. You'll also need to make sure they are adequately hydrated.

Jaundice and Breast-Feeding

Sometimes, doctors will refer to jaundice in week-old nursing babies as *breast-feeding jaundice*. They'll call jaundice in older babies *breast-milk jaundice,* a form of the disease that occurs in over one-third of all breast-fed babies and can last up to three months. Don't let the name put you off. Studies have shown that breast-feeding is actually good for babies with jaundice, because breast milk is rich in fluid and calories, which seems to improve liver and intestinal functioning. However, in some cases, breast-feeding does mean that one or both babies aren't getting enough nutrition or hydration, which can drive the bilirubin levels up. If this is your situation, you might need to supplement breast-feedings with bottle-feedings of nutritional supplements and/or hydrating liquids.

Myths about Jaundice

Since jaundice is such a common ailment among newborns—both premature and full-term—you may already have heard many parents discussing this condition. If you hear that "it's no big deal" or "lots of babies get it," you're hearing correctly. But don't believe the person who tells you that sunshine or natural light will cure jaundice. Sunbathing outdoors is bad for newborns, whose tender skin can't take the prolonged exposure.

When Can They Come Home?

Every doctor has slightly different standards for deciding when a baby—or two babies!—is ready to be released from the hospital. Generally, though, here's what we expect:

- The babies should be able to maintain their body temperatures at room temperature.
- They have to be taking all feedings by mouth, either through the bottle or through the breast.
- If born before 34 weeks' gestation, the babies should be gaining 20 to 30 grams a day for three to five days.
- Premature babies who are not being medicated for respiratory problems should be apnea-free for four to seven days.
- Premature babies who *are* being medicated for respiratory problems should be apnea-free for three days—and their parents should be prepared to do home apnea monitoring.

Postpartum Depression

These days, the term *depression*—whether postpartum or "regular"—gets tossed around rather often. It can be hard to know when the term refers to a serious condition that needs special treatment and when it more casually signifies having a temporary hard time. Just about every new mother feels tired, overwhelmed, and pessimistic at least *some* of the time, and multiple moms have an even harder row to hoe, particularly if one or both of their children were premature or have other complications. So are their down times depression or just the "baby blues"?

Interestingly, postpartum depression is far less common in cultures where mothers are not left alone after birth but are instead surrounded by the female members of the culture at all times. This suggests that whatever the medical components of postpartum depression, a strong support system and a breakdown of the isolation common to most mothers of newborns can go a long way toward easing the hard times that can follow a birth.

You May Have Mild Postpartum Depression If You Feel Unusually

- prone to crying;
- pessimistic;
- anxious;
- short-tempered;
- restless.

So how seriously should you take your down times—and how do you know? Experts have identified three types of postpartum depression:

1. a mild, passing depression, often called "the baby blues" or "maternity blues," common to 50 to 70 percent of all twin moms;
2. classic postpartum depression, marked by more serious symptoms, found in 10 to 15 percent of all mothers of twins;
3. depression marked by psychosis, which is extremely rare.

It may be hard to know how to diagnose yourself—especially at 3:00 A.M., when the house is a mess, your babies are crying, and you're feeling particularly helpless and hopeless. Here are some checklists to help you distinguish between mild and classic postpartum depression.

Some doctors suspect that this type of depression is caused by altered tryptophan levels after birth. (Tryptophan is a hormone that helps the brain's neurotransmitters process emotion and cope with stress.) Others think that these feelings are simply caused by lack of sleep. Women who suffer from this type of mild depression usually feel its effects within ten days of giving birth. If you're experiencing the baby blues, you should be feeling better a few days after that.

Obviously, any new mother—especially a new mother of twins—will feel at least *some* of these things at least *some* of the time. But if

You May Have Classic Postpartum Depression if You

- find yourself crying for several minutes at a time, three or more times a week;
- worry unduly about your ability to care for your babies, your other children's safety, your partner's interest in you, or some other aspect of your life;
- fantasize frequently (everyone fantasizes occasionally) about leaving your family;
- have frequent thoughts of suicide, illness, or accidental death;
- feel an unusual degree of anger, envy, or indifference toward your partner and/or children;
- feel convinced that you'll never be able to go back to work or otherwise resume your premultiple life;
- are consistently too exhausted to play with your children or to enjoy any of your prepregnancy activities;
- feel generally "down," "flat," or "blank";
- have trouble sleeping, even when your babies are asleep;
- are losing an unusual amount of weight;
- have no interest in food or what seems like an excessive interest in food.

your sense of "hopelessness and helplessness"—the classic description of depression—seems to pervade your life more often than not, you may need to take some steps to address this problem. You're particularly at risk for classic postpartum depression if you:

- were ever diagnosed with depression or another psychiatric condition before your pregnancy;
- had a complication during your pregnancy;
- felt that the birth "took you by surprise," especially if the delivery was complicated;
- have had to cope with an additional strain, such as the death or severe illness of a family member; an economic strain; a problem with your or your partner's job; emotional difficulties experienced by your other children, such as jealousy of the new babies; and the like.

My patient Shirla had a tough bout with postpartum depression. As she explains it, "I had been waiting ten years to have a baby—and I was so thrilled to have twins. Yet when the babies had finally come and I was settled back at home, I found myself overcome with all sorts of feelings I didn't expect. Everyone said, 'Oh, it's just the baby blues; you'll get over it.' And I was sure I *couldn't* be feeling as bad as I *thought* I was feeling, because didn't I finally have everything I'd always wanted? Still, I found myself thinking a *lot* about just leaving everything behind, just getting on a bus and going somewhere I'd never been before, and finding a little house somewhere and living alone. I didn't think of myself as depressed—just tired. Then one day I saw myself in the mirror, and I thought, 'Who *is* that miserable-looking woman?' Suddenly it hit me how long it had been since *anything* had made me smile—even the twins.

"Eventually, I went to see a therapist, who wanted to put me on antidepressants. I said, 'But I'm still nursing!' She said, 'Would you rather breast-feed your babies or be able to smile at them?' After two agonizing weeks of soul-searching, I weaned the twins and went on the meds. Things *did* get better, slowly but surely—I'm sure because I also decided to go back to work, which I'd thought I was going to put off for another two or three years. I used to feel ashamed of what happened to me, but now I think it was my way of giving myself a wake-up call. The decisions I had made just weren't working—it was time to make a change. Now I can enjoy my children, *and* my husband, *and* my job, without feeling like I'm selling everybody short."

Coping with Postpartum Depression

Many multiple moms have a hard time knowing whether life is tough just because it *is*—two children! no sleep! changing identities! no sleep!—or if their hard times are a sign of depression that needs to be treated: through therapy, a multiple moms' support group, medication, or some combination of the three. To complicate the diagnosis further, some women are suffering from hypothyroidism—low thyroid function—after birth, and all *they* need is to take thyroid supplements for a while.

In my own opinion, it's always worth reaching out for support and comfort—especially at the times when it seems most difficult to do so. If you're having a hard time coping with your new life as a multiple mom, turn to your partner, friends, and family for support. Read a book like *Mothering the New Mother,* by Sally Placksin, or have your partner read it. Check out the possibility of a multiple parents' support group, or even a singleton mothers' group. Find a therapist to talk to: Even if you're *not* suffering from depression, you might benefit from some counseling and support as you adjust to your new identity and the unexpected demands on your time and energy.

If your sense of hopelessness does not recede, you might want to explore the possibilities of antidepressants. Some antidepressants do permit a woman to continue nursing, although these often have more side effects. You may also decide that your babies are better served by a happier, calmer mother than by the nutritional benefits of breast milk.

Typically, the symptoms of classic postpartum depression tend to recur about 12 months after they've finally disappeared. So if you are taking medication, you may be asked to continue for 18 months. If you're seeing a therapist, make sure that he or she is available for your "one-year anniversary."

One final piece of advice: Find a way to let your partner in on what you're going through. Schedule some couples counseling or make a regular date—*without* the babies—to share a quiet half hour together. If you're a single parent, find a way to draw on friends and family for support during this crucial time. (That's actually good advice even if you're *not* a single parent.) Feeling depressed and feeling isolated often make for a tight little vicious circle, exacerbated by the fact that it *is* hard to connect to other adults when you're caring for two or more little children. If you can reach out past the isolation, though, you may find new comfort from others—and a new strength within yourself.

You and Your Family

You're about to take your two new children home from the hospital—and change your family forever. Maybe these are your first children; maybe you've got older ones at home. Either way, your family has probably never cared for multiples before.

Remember, it's not only your twins who need to be monitored. If you can take some time—even a few minutes—to think about other members of your family, you'll all be more likely to handle the demands of your new situation with patience and grace.

19.

Now That They're Here:
Adapting to Your New Life

⚜

This can be a challenging time, in which you struggle to recover your prepregnancy levels of strength and health while caring for not one but *two* new babies—as well as for any other children who may be waiting for you at home. If I were going to give you only one piece of advice to help get you through, it would be: *Be patient.* Easier said than done, especially when you're feeling absolutely exhausted and two hungry children are crying in your arms. But I promise, this too will pass. And amidst the fatigue and the craziness, there are also moments of wonder and joy.

"I never expected being a parent would change me so much," Miriam says, somewhat ruefully. "It hasn't really made me more patient, or more tolerant, or any of the things that I might have expected. What it has done is made me more . . . appreciative, I guess would be the word. Every so often, I'll just *stop,* right in the middle of whatever I'm doing, and I just pay attention, in a way I never did before. I feel like I really *notice* Ira, and the kids, and the other things in my life that make me happy—just this one quiet moment, and then the craziness starts again. But those moments make everything else worthwhile."

Taking Stock

When you and your twins are finally home from the hospital, you and your family might want to take a moment to see how everyone is doing. In the hustle and bustle of *two* new arrivals, a lot can get lost in the shuffle. Some families like to set aside a special weekly time— Sunday evening, say, or a special meal over the weekend—just to keep up with all the changes.

Here are examples of some of the family issues that might come up in those first few weeks after you get home:

The Mother

- Are you getting *any* sleep? Can anyone help you get more?
- Are you eating well? Remember, you need to keep your strength up—especially if you're breast-feeding. If you're not eating, who can help prepare food that you might like?
- Are you feeling comfortable feeding and caring for your newborns?
- Do you have a list of resource people who can help you cope?
- Have you managed to establish a household routine?

The Father/The Partner

- Have you found special parts of the child-care routine that are "just for you"? Particularly when the mother is breast-feeding and/or when the partner is working full-time, it can be hard to make special "Daddy/co-parent" time, but I urge you to find some routine or ritual that you and your children can share, right from the beginning. You'll be surprised at what a difference it makes as your relationship continues to grow and develop.
- Have you been able to take time off from work—paternity leave or at least an extra few days around the homecoming? Our society is often sadly neglectful of the father's role in child-rearing, but again, any time you can take now, at the beginning, will

make a big difference in both you and your partner's sense of your participation.

- Are *you* getting the emotional support you need? Adding two babies to a household can be stressful at best, overwhelming at worst. A lot of the focus may be on the mother, especially if she's breast-feeding and/or recovering from a C-section or a difficult birth. Make sure you don't lose *yourself* in the shuffle.

The Couple

- Have you found at least a little time to talk to each other each day? Amidst the demands of two crying newborns, the emotional needs of two adults can easily get shoved aside. But you two are a team, and you need each other to get through all the extraordinary demands of that first year of twin babyhood.
- Do you have—or can you get—support for yourself as a couple? Do you have child care—a paid sitter, a cooperative relative— who will take the babies for an hour, an afternoon, an evening, so that the two of you can have some quiet time together? Although there will be lots of demands on your time and energy, can you make a place for some couple rituals?

Other Children

- Are your other children secure in their place in the family, or are they feeling a bit shoved aside? Are they acting out, getting sick, or finding themselves in other kinds of trouble that require extra parental attention?
- Can you make some special time—even if it's only ten minutes a day—that each child knows is his or hers alone?
- Is it possible to find some special new privileges that go with being "the oldest," some new rewards for helping out with two new little siblings?

Choosing Your Pediatrician

One of the most dramatic changes that mark the transition from prenatal care to early childhood is the switch from ob/gyn to pediatrician. Just as you had to balance lots of factors in your search for an obstetrician, so you must keep lots of factors in mind as you select the doctor who will care for your new children.

Ideally, you'll choose your pediatrician during the pregnancy. For a singleton pregnancy, parents often wait as late as 35 weeks, but if you're carrying twins, I suggest you start a lot earlier than that. As you well know by now, twin pregnancies are marked by a higher incidence of preterm labor and by a greater likelihood that your ob/gyn will prescribe bed rest or even a hospital stay. I've known some families who have done the search by phone, from the mother's hospital bed. One husband I knew faithfully made the initial visit to three or four pediatricians, reported back to his wife, on home bed rest, and then asked each doctor if he or she would be willing to visit his wife at home. Needless to say, the doctor willing to make the house call won!

Lots of new parents rely on friends, relatives, and neighbors for recommendations, but I'd advise caution, for two reasons. First, people's child-rearing styles can vary wildly, even if they're soul mates in every other respect. (You may have already noticed this as you and your husband or partner work through your various preparations and decisions.) If you don't like a friend's way of raising her kids, you're not likely to be very happy with her pediatrician either.

Second, unless your friend also has twins, you've got slightly different needs in that regard. You want a pediatrician with a lot of experience dealing with twins and other high-risk infants. If your babies have to spend some time in the hospital before going home, you'll probably want your pediatrician to be the one to care for them or at least to be involved in their care—so you need a doctor with privileges at your hospital.

Here are some questions you might ask the doctors you're considering choosing for your pediatrician:

- How many twins have you treated?
- How soon after our twins are born would you like to see them?
- How often do you want to see well babies?
- What's the usual routine at a well-baby visit? How will that apply to our twins?

- Suppose our babies are premature? How would you adjust your scheduling and treatment?
- What do you think are the differences between treating twins and caring for singletons?
- Our philosophy concerning medication is _____. What's your opinion of that approach?
- Our philosophy concerning child care is _____. How does that fit in with your approach?
- What's your policy on calls to the office with questions?
- What happens if we call after office hours?
- What's your policy on emergencies?
- Who else might end up caring for our babies?

What's Important to You?

One of the hardest parts of bringing two babies home from the hospital is that all of a sudden, *everything* seems important. You've got children to feed, diaper, and bathe; bills to pay; groceries to buy; meals to cook; housework to do; let alone other children to care for and jobs to attend. In this hectic atmosphere, there often seems to be no chance to actually *enjoy* your children, let alone any time for parents to communicate with each other, to reach out to friends and relatives, or to have a moment to themselves.

I have two suggestions:

1. FIGURE OUT WHAT'S TRULY IMPORTANT TO YOU AND *PUT THAT BEFORE ALL ELSE.* If a clean house is tops on your list, then go ahead and make that your top priority. But perhaps you'd rather let the dust pile up in the living room and enjoy a hot bath, a quiet half hour with your partner, a few moments of playing with your babies. Likewise, money in the bank may seem like the thing you need most to get through the next several years of family life. But perhaps some of that money would be better spent on a sitter, a housekeeper, take-out meals, or some other way of buying a little time to refresh and recharge.

This can seem like difficult advice to follow in those frantic first few months. You may feel as though you're running faster than you ever have before, just to stay in place. But if you can, take a step back and think through your priorities to be sure you're not just going on

My Patients Tell What They Learned to Let Go of

Natalie: For one whole year, there was no more homemade *anything* in our house. Before, Janet used to bake—cookies, cake, sometimes pie—and I would get into making vegetable stews and soups and casseroles. After the twins came, there were lots more cans and frozen foods in our kitchen—and lots more take-out containers in our trash!

Sarah: Both Philip and I used to be very good about staying in touch with our families—birthday cards, birthday calls, long chats with my sisters, leisurely family days with Philip's older brother and his kids. Now that time goes for our own family.

Marsha: I exercise a *lot* less. I hate to admit it, but I do.

Rosario: I wouldn't say the house is a *mess*. But it's not as neat as I think it should be, let's just put it that way.

automatic pilot or giving lots of time to tasks that really might be allowed to slide.

2. FIGURE OUT WHAT OTHER PEOPLE CAN DO, AND THEN *DELEGATE THOSE TASKS TO THEM.* If you've got other children at home, now's the time for them to pitch in and help with all those household chores that they're finally old enough to do. If you've got friends and neighbors who have offered to lend a hand, see if you can pass along your shopping list, ask them to supply you with frozen meals, or schedule some baby-sitting time.

Let me repeat once again: It can be hard to reach out for help in our individualistic, do-it-yourself society. But for parents of multiples, accepting and even asking for support is absolutely crucial. For hundreds of thousands of years, human societies have raised children in large, extended families, with lots of adults around to care for whatever children happened to cross their path. It's only recently that we've expected one stay-at-home adult and one working parent to care for two, three, or more children all by themselves. Unless you're very lucky, you probably won't be able to re-create the child-care conditions of an

African village or a medieval English hamlet. But you *can* schedule regular or irregular baby-sitting dates with willing friends and relatives; ask neighbors to help you shop and carpool your other children; make a list of chores that some outsider might do, and have a suggestion ready when a friend says, "How can I help?"

Organized Support Systems

Let me put in another word on behalf of Mothers of Twins clubs and other similar support groups. Although they don't work for everybody, many of my patients have found them to be lifesavers. See Chapter 4 and the Resources section at the end of this book for some suggestions on how to hook up with these support systems.

Survival Tips

Finally, here are my own personal survival suggestions, culled from my own years as a multiple mom as well as from the stories my patients have told me. You may find none, some, or all of them helpful—use or adapt them any way that fits into your own personal situation. You also might start making your own personal list of survival tips based on suggestions from friends, family, your own doctor, or your support group.

- **Have a family bulletin board.** Whenever anyone in the family thinks of something that needs to be done or remembered, they can make a note. If you get the kind of bulletin board that uses dry-erase markers, you can "wipe the slate clean" each night and start fresh each morning with such notes as *Last feeding at 8:00 P.M.—next feeding, midnight!* or *Call sitter for Saturday afternoon!*
- **Get the twins sleeping in their own beds as soon as possible.**
- **Do all you can to get your twins on a sleeping schedule.** By the third week, it's realistic—though not always possible—to hope that your twins will be sleeping more at night than during the day. Even if you're not getting any *more* sleep, you'll feel less isolated and crazy if the sleep you are getting is at night rather than during the day.

How My Patients Created Support Systems

Zoe: We really pulled Rosie into our family in a way that we'd never wanted to do before. I think we hit her at a vulnerable time in her own life—she's 45, and she was just starting to realize that she'd probably never have kids of her own. So I think it worked out well for all of us—she got closer to Sean and Lissa, and we had some support that we really needed.

Natalie: We have these next-door neighbors who had a one-year-old and a three-year-old when our twins were just babies. We didn't really even know each other all that well—but we worked out this system where they'd take all the kids one weekend afternoon, and we'd get them all the following Saturday or Sunday. The on-duty day was pretty overwhelming—but that free afternoon was a treasure.

Miriam: Ira and I really leaned on our mothers during that first year. His mother was great about coming over for an afternoon if we'd give her a ride both ways, or for an evening if we'd let her stay over. My mother was willing to have us drop the kids off for an overnight or even a weekend, once they had stopped nursing. I didn't expect to enjoy so much contact with them—and I wouldn't say we didn't pay a price—but they both do love being grandmothers, I'll give them that.

Marsha: What I missed most was talking to someone who *wasn't* involved with the kids. I'd always been close to my friend Celia, but after the babies came, I found I was really *hungry* for adult conversation. Celia and I started chatting on the phone a lot more than we ever had—sometimes about the kids, sometimes about other things. I can't tell you how much that meant.

- **Use baby monitors.** Many new parents find themselves anxious about leaving their newborns alone in their room, even for a few minutes. If you carry a baby monitor with you at all times, leaving the companion monitor with your twins, you can always reassure yourself that your babies are breathing normally and doing fine.
- **Keep talking to your partner.** If one of you is working and the other is staying home with the kids, that can be fertile ground

for miscommunication. The working parent fantasizes about the lovely, peaceful time at home, while the stay-at-home grits her teeth at the sound of crying babies and wonders when they'll *ever* get onto a regular feeding schedule. It might sound mechanical, but I find it helpful to make a rule: At the end of each day, each partner gets ten minutes to talk while the other listens. (You could cut it down to five minutes each if you're feeling *really* sleep-deprived!) You can use that time to complain about problems, crow over triumphs, or simply to share information.

- **Make special time for your other children.** A special bedtime song or cuddle for younger children; a weekly half-hour walk to the donut stand for older kids; a family council every Sunday night—there are lots of creative ways to remind your older kids that they count too.

The Ups and Downs of Multiple Parenthood

As I think back to the lessons I've learned from multiple parenthood, it's the words of my patient Marsha that resonate the loudest: "You *can* have it all. Just not all at the same time." For me and the women I've treated, multiple parenthood has often meant giving up on some cherished dreams—or at least postponing them for a while. It's also meant cutting back on activities and relationships that once meant the world to us—or at least putting them on hold.

On the other hand, for me and my patients, multiple parenthood has been an amazing journey in which we've learned more about ourselves—and what really matters to us—than we'd ever thought possible. Taking care of two or three infants; watching them grow into active, healthy children; helping them discover themselves and their abilities; cuddling with them in the morning and reading stories to them at night—these activities bring a joy and a satisfaction like no other.

It's also clear to me that every parent's journey into multiple parenthood is unique. I wish you luck and joy on your journey.

Resources

Organizations

These nationwide organizations for parents of multiples can put you in touch with local chapters. Their websites are sources of information and support.

The National Organization of Mothers of Twins Clubs, Inc. (NOMOTC)
Executive Office
P.O. Box 438
Thompsons Station, TN 37179-0438
Tel: (615) 595-0936
Referral line: (877) 540-2200
Email: NOMOTC@aol.com
Website: www.nomotc.org

The Triplet Connection
P.O. Box 99571
Stockton, CA 95209
Tel: (209) 474-0885
Fax: (209) 474-9243
Email: tc@tripletconnection.org
Website: www.tripletconnection.org

Major medical associations you might contact:

American College of Obstetricians and Gynecologists (ACOG)
409 Twelfth Street S.W.
P.O. Box 96920
Washington, D.C. 20090-6920
Tel: (202) 863-2518
Email: resources@acog.org
Website: www.acog.org
Offers a wide range of resources and information with excellent patient education material and has a list of members in your area.

American Society of Reproductive Medicine (ASRM)
1209 Montgomery Highway
Birmingham, AL 35216-2809
Tel: (205) 978-5000
Fax: (205) 978-5005
Email: asrm@asrm.org
Website: www.asrm.org
For information on infertility and assisted reproductive technologies, including excellent patient fact sheets.

Society for Maternal-Fetal Medicine
409 Twelfth Street, S.W.
Washington, D.C. 20024
Tel: (202) 863-2476
Fax: (202) 554-1132
Email: info@smfm.org
Website: www.smfm.org
Lists of subspecialists, research.

Other organizations of interest:

Mothers of Supertwins (MOST)
P.O. Box 951
Brentwood, NY 11717-0627
Tel: (631) 859-1110
Email: info@MOSTonline.org
Website: www.mostonline.org
An international support network dedicated to families with triplets, quads, or quints.

The International Twins Association
6898 Channel Road NE
Minneapolis, MN 55432
Tel: (612) 571-3022
Email: ITAconvention@aol.com
Website: www.intltwins.org
A non-profit organization dedicated to promoting twins' welfare.

The Center for Study of Multiple Birth (CSMB)
333 E. Superior Street, Suite 464
Chicago, IL 60611
Tel: (312) 908-7532
Fax: (312) 908-8500
Email: lgk395@nwu.edu
Website: www.multiplebirth.com
Charity organized to support research in multiple birth and also help parents with the special issues their multiples may face.

International Society for Twin Studies (ISTS)
Website: www.ists.qimr.edu.au
An international nonprofit organization whose purpose is to further research and public education in all fields related to twins. Twin Research *is its official journal.*

The Twins Foundation
P.O. Box 6043
Providence, RI 02940-6043
Tel: (401) 729-1000
Fax: (401) 751-4642
Email: twins@twinsfoundation.com
Website: www.twinsfoundation.com
A nonprofit membership and research information organization, includes a National twins registry and a quarterly newsletter, The Twins Foundation Newsletter.

Twins Services Consulting
Email: twinservices@juno.com
Website: www.twinservices.org

An excellent resource for loss in multiple pregnancy is:

Center for Loss in Multiple Birth (CLIMB), Inc.
c/o Jean Kollantai
P.O. Box 91377
Anchorage, AK 99509
Tel: (907) 222-5321
Email: climb@pobox.alaska.net or webmaster@climb-support.org
Website: www.climb-support.org

An organization dedicated to complicated or high risk pregnancy support is:

Sidelines National Support Network
Sideline High Risk Pregnancy Support National Office
P.O. Box 1808
Laguna Beach, CA 92652
Tel: (888) 447-4754
Fax: (949) 497-5598
Email: sidelines@sidelines.org
Website: www.sidelines.org
The muliples group coordinator can be accessed through their excellent website.

Twin to Twin Transfusion Syndrome Foundation
411 Longbeach Parkway
Bay Village, OH 44140
Tel: (440) 899-8887
Email: info@tttsfoundation.org
Website: www.tttsfoundation.org
A nonprofit group that supports parents affected by pregnancies with TTTS.

Twin Hope, Inc.
2592 West 14th Street
Cleveland, OH 44113
Tel: (502) 243-2110 24 hr. hotline
Email: twinhope@twinhope.com
Website: www.twinhope.com
An organization helping families affected by TTTS and other complications of multiple pregnancies.

Publications

Our Newsletter (quarterly)
Center for Loss in Multiple Birth, Inc. (CLIMB)
Tel: (907) 746-6123

Twin Lines
Twin Hope, Inc.

TWINS magazine (published 6 times each year)
5350 South Roslyn Street
Suite 400
Englewood, CO 80111
Tel: (800) 328-3211
Website: www.twinsmagazine.com

The Twins Foundation Newsletter (quarterly)
The Twins Foundation
P.O. Box 6043
Providence, RI 02940
Tel: (401) 729-1000

Twins Research (journal)
International Society for Twin Studies (ISTS)

Additional Web Sites

www.motherisk.org—*for information on potential risks to a developing fetus*
www.obgyn.net—*for general gynecological information*
www.resolve.org—*for information on infertility*
www.reprotox.org—*for information on environmental hazards to human re-production*

Maternity Needs

Talk to your doctor or local twins/triplets club to find local sources of products for multiple moms and infants. Here are a few additional suggestions:

Support Hose and Undergarments
About Babies, Inc.
1818 Blue Gitt Ave.
Clare, MI 48617
Tel: (800) 383-3068
Email: contact@aboutbabiesinc.com
Website: www.aboutbabiesinc.com
A mail order and online catalog with supportive undergarments and stockings for pregnancy.

Medi Support Hose
76 Seegers Road
Arlington Heights, IL 60005
Tel: (800) 633-6334
Prescription-only support hose (support hose also available at retail level).

Jobst Support Hose
P.O. Box 653
Toledo, OH 43697
Tel: (800) 537-1063
Prescription-only support hose and maternity girdles (support hose also available at retail level).

Breast–Feeding

International Lactation Consultant Association (ILCA)
1500 Sunday Drive, Suite 102
Raleigh, NC 27607
Tel: (919) 787-5181
Fax: (919) 787-4916
Email: ilca@erols.com
Website: www.users.erols.com/ilca/
Has information about lactation consultants, and a publication list.

La Leche League International
1400 N. Meacham Road
Schaumburg, IL 60173-4048
Tel: (800) LA-LECHE
Website: www.lalecheleague.org
Wide variety of information on breast-feeding, as well as nursing items, including nursing pillows, breast shells for women with inverted nipples, nursing pads, nursing stool (to aid posture), heat pads, lanolin cream, milk freezer bags, and baby cups for infants too small to suck properly.

Medela
Tel: (800) 435-8316
Website: www.medela.com
Breast pumps and nursing aids available at retail level; toll-free number helps customer find nearest outlet and/or consultant.

Index